"Courtney Worley and Michael Nadorff, both seasoned sleep experts, offer a clear, compassionate guide to understanding and managing nightmares. As a clinician, I value the practical self-check questions and step-by-step strategies. Whether for yourself or a loved one, this accessible and well-structured book is an empowering toolkit to help you take control of your sleep and find relief."

> —**Yishan Xu, PhD,** adjunct faculty at Stanford Sleep Medicine Center, chair of the Public Education Committee of the Society of Behavioral Sleep Medicine, and host of the *Deep into Sleep* podcast

"The toolkit includes practical steps to deal with nightmares and sleep problems related to nightmares. The good news: Research has shown that the techniques outlined in the book are very helpful—even for persons who had nightmares for years. As it is valid for many topics, if you take action using this toolkit, something positive will happen."

> —**Michael Schredl, PhD,** head of research for the sleep laboratory at the Central Institute of Mental Health in Mannheim, Germany; and author of *Analyzing a Long Dream Series*

"Many people are surprised to learn that nightmares can be treated without medication. This book is packed with useful tools that research has shown to be useful in therapy. The ideas are solid, and could really help people who want to work on their nightmares on their own. It offers a sense of hope and direction for something that can often feel overwhelming or out of control."

> —**Kristi E. Pruiksma, PhD, DBSM,** associate professor in the department of psychiatry and behavioral sciences at the University of Texas Health Science Center at San Antonio, licensed clinical psychologist, and diplomat of behavioral sleep medicine

"Worley and Nadorff have crafted a must-have workbook for anyone who struggles with nightmares. They have distilled their decades of expertise into a comprehensive book that explains the basics of nightmares, as well as evidence-based treatment approaches for nightmares and insomnia. Purchase this book today and transform your life by getting better sleep!"

> —**S. Justin Thomas, PhD, DBSM, FSBSM,** director of the UAB Behavioral Sleep Medicine Program, and former president of the Society of Behavioral Sleep Medicine

"*The Nightmare and Sleep Disorder Toolkit* guides the reader toward understanding their sleep problems and using skills to reduce or resolve them. At each step, Worley and Nadorff explain the science and theories behind sleep problems, and how each skill works to address them. Readers will appreciate the accessible explanations and having this accompanying guide and resource as they work toward achieving better, more restorative sleep."

>—**Jennifer Fanning, PhD,** clinical psychologist, and faculty at McLean Hospital and Harvard Medical School

"*The Nightmare and Sleep Disorder Toolkit* is a valuable resource for those struggling with sleep disturbances related to nightmares. It offers practical strategies and exercises to understand and address the causes of sleep problems. The workbook provides a clear and structured approach, empowering readers to take control of their sleep health and improve their well-being. Highly recommended for those seeking effective solutions to enhance sleep quality and overcome nightmares."

>—**Kathryn Hansen, BS, CPC, CPMA,** healthcare consultant at Integration Consultants, LLC; author of *Fundamental of Sleep Technology*; and executive director of the Society of Behavioral Sleep Medicine

The Nightmare & Sleep Disorder Toolkit

A Workbook to Help You Get Some Rest
Using Imagery Rehearsal Therapy & Other
Evidence-Based Approaches

Courtney Worley, PhD, MPH | Michael R. Nadorff, PhD

New Harbinger Publications, Inc.

Publisher's Note

This publication is designed to provide accurate and authoritative information in regard to the subject matter covered. It is sold with the understanding that the publisher is not engaged in rendering psychological, financial, legal, or other professional services. If expert assistance or counseling is needed, the services of a competent professional should be sought.

NEW HARBINGER PUBLICATIONS is a registered trademark of New Harbinger Publications, Inc.

New Harbinger Publications is an employee-owned company.

Copyright © 2025 by Courtney Worley and Michael R. Nadorff
New Harbinger Publications, Inc.
5720 Shattuck Avenue
Oakland, CA 94609
www.newharbinger.com

All Rights Reserved

Cover design by Amy Shoup

Acquired by Elizabeth Hollis Hansen

Edited by Jennifer Holder

Library of Congress Cataloging-in-Publication Data on file

TK

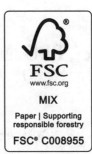

Printed in the United States of America

27	26	25							
10	9	8	7	6	5	4	3	2	1

First Printing

Contents

	Foreword	V
CHAPTER 1	Sleep and Nightmare Basics	1
CHAPTER 2	Measure Sleep and Nightmares to Track Progress	11
CHAPTER 3	Treatment Elements and Methods for Nightmares	25
CHAPTER 4	Choosing a Path for Nightmare Recovery	37
CHAPTER 5	Sleep Hygiene	55
CHAPTER 6	Relaxation	75
CHAPTER 7	Visualization	89
CHAPTER 8	Exposure and Rescription	101
CHAPTER 9	Sleep Restriction and Stimulus Control	117
CHAPTER 10	Lucid Dreaming and Lucidity Checks	125
CHAPTER 11	Cognitive Restructuring	133
CHAPTER 12	Relapse Prevention	145
	References	155

Foreword

Nightmares have only recently become a major topic of discussion in psychology and medicine. The group I worked with for my first nightmare treatment research project wanted to demonstrate that lucid dreaming is a highly potent technique for overcoming frequent nightmares. We recruited our "subjects" using the media and colleagues at the University Clinic of Vienna. Our participants hardly understood that frequent or recurring nightmares are a phenomenon that could be overcome!

Nightmares were considered a matter of fate—unusual, threatening and terrifying as they are—and many people wouldn't even consider mentioning nightmares to a practitioner.

At that time, Barry Krakow's approach to nightmares, Imagery Rehearsal Therapy (IRT) already existed. He had just published his first peer-reviewed publications about the effectiveness of IRT as a potential cure for nightmares.

Post-traumatic stress disorder (PTSD) has only been recognized as a diagnosis since the Vietnam War, and acceptance of the effect PTSD can have on sleep, dreams and nightmares only recently is even newer still.

In short, nightmare treatment research is still a field of pioneer work, and we learn more about it and its potential correlations with other mental health challenges every day.

This book is a notable step toward further enhancing our ability to treat nightmares and improve the lives of the millions of people who struggle with them. Its uniqueness lies in the fact that it's a product of two different experts—one focused on PTSD and the other on non-trauma nightmares—who see the world of nightmares just a bit differently.

Dr. Courtney Worley has worked in intensive trauma and behavioral sleep medicine clinics in the US Department of Veterans Affairs. She was a lead trainer on Written Exposure Therapy, an empirically supported treatment for PTSD. She became interested in nightmares through finding that even after concluding trauma treatment, nightmares often persisted. This led to her incorporating treatments such as Imagery Rehearsal Therapy; Exposure, Relaxation, and Rescriptioning Therapy; and Lucid Dreaming Therapy. She still believes strongly in the importance of exposure therapy for many individuals and typically includes exposure in her practice of treating nightmares.

The second author, Dr. Michael Nadorff, views the treatment of nightmares a bit differently. While he believes that exposure is sometimes required, he has had a lot of success without using it and believes that nightmares can often be treated without it. He is one of the first psychologists to discover a connection between nightmare frequency and suicidal ideation and suicidality. He ascertained that it is particularly the younger crowd affected by experiencing frequent or recurrent nightmares, potentially revealing that there is more behind nightmares, e.g. suicidality – a great danger to children and adolescents. He is a true pioneer and dedicated researcher who has investigated how to change, solve, and transform nightmares so that even the underlying reasons for them can potentially solve themselves by resolving the nightmares.

The world of psychology is lucky that these pioneers are emerging to reveal the secrets of nightmares and the benefits of nightmare treatment. The fact that they view the nightmare world slightly differently gives the reader a unique opportunity to hear both experts discuss multiple theories and treatment options and then pick the path that speaks most to them. It gives a more complete view of the treatment options and rationale than would be obtained otherwise.

This book is a hands-on guide for nightmare treatment at home, when the nightmare might haunt you and make you lose— or even avoid—valuable hours of sleep, which restore us on all levels, but particularly our mental well-being.

It is also a scientific, state-of-the-art book on methods that are carefully selected and introduced to the reader: basic sleep hygiene and sleep coaching, relaxation, visualization, exposure and rescription, Imagery Rehearsal Therapy, and Lucid Dreaming Therapy.

With this book the reader can start to influence and eventually overcome their nightmares. They will also be able to better understand why nightmares might occur and even what treasures they might hold for our personal growth.

This book provides an excellent overview of cutting-edge theories, research, and approaches to nightmares. Therefore, it is to be recommended to nightmare sufferers as well as their peers, their caregivers, psychologists, teachers, and social workers. Anybody who has something to do with nightmares or has the slightest interest in the topic will gain deep knowledge about them and take away personal solutions tailored to their specific needs.

The book provides and introduction to the best possible approaches to nightmares that are currently known. It is well-written and well-structured and guides you through a murky topic, making it accessible. It shines a light through the darkness that nightmares frequently entail.

Choose any one of the well-explained and described techniques, and soon you will understand why your "other side" had to develop these nightly horrors for you to become aware of the important issues hidden in your subconscious.

Experiencing the occasional nightmare is considered normal, but having to bear them several times per week can negatively affect you. I still remember one of my former clients who participated in our nightmare treatment research project for patients with PTSD. Even though she took an enormous amount of medication intended to reduce her nightmares, she still experienced several nightmares per week and the sleep loss that came with them. This was highly instrumental in encouraging her to face her nightmares and sleep problems. In a few weeks she succeeded in changing and overcoming her nightmares.

The scars the life-forming and sometimes life-threatening events and relationships that can inform our nightmares leave on our souls cannot be undone, but they can be understood, changed, and eventually overcome. Addressing your nightmares allows for some light into the darkness of one's nightly experiences—once explained as demons and dragons, today understood as unfinished business, or, as we say in Gestalt therapy, longing for closure. Just reading this book will help you move in the right direction.

When you pick up this book, maybe even with a trained companion, if you can, you can look forward to an unburdened life and— as my client told me after several years of being able to change her nightmares into interesting dreams—get a new life without threats and demons, night and day!

—*Brigitte Holzinger*

CHAPTER 1

Sleep and Nightmare Basics

Nightmares are universal experiences. Almost everyone experiences a nightmare at one point or another. Some people, like you, have nightmares that can become a recurrent problem lasting years or even decades. Nightmares cause problems not just when they are happening, but in other parts of your sleep cycle. In waking hours, you might notice fatigue, sleepiness, irritability, and problems with memory and concentration. If you are struggling with nightmares on a regular basis (weekly or more frequently), whether due to trauma or posttraumatic stress disorder (PTSD) or a nightmare disorder, or there is no clear event causing the nightmares, this book was written for you.

The Fundamentals of Sleep

Sleep is universal. Every human has a biological need for sleep, though sleep needs vary across the lifespan. For instance, infants typically need fourteen to seventeen hours of sleep per day and children need nine to twelve hours. In adulthood, we need six to eight hours a night on average. But that does not mean we get that much sleep. Older adults often find it difficult to sleep enough, not because they don't need it, but because they encounter changes in sleep architecture and often have medical issues that disturb sleep.

We all need sleep to survive and thrive, so if you're struggling with chronic nightmares, you're probably not getting the sleep you need. We want to help you find a balance of sleep that improves your quality of life. In treatment, we focus on *quality* of sleep over quantity.

Think about what good, quality sleep would mean for you. Does it mean having fewer nightmares or being able to sleep until you naturally wake up in the morning? What would it mean for your performance or mood the next day?

If I was sleeping well, I would... _____

_____

_____

_____

There are lots of ways to define good sleep. Everyone has different goals. In this workbook, we want you to meet *your* goals.

Sleep Structure

We spend about a third of our lives sleeping. Sleep and wake usually occur in a regular cycle: the average adult sleeps between six to eight hours, usually at night, and is awake for the other sixteen to eighteen hours. This is called the *circadian rhythm*, (*circadian* is Latin for "about a day") and it keeps us in sync with the 24-hour day. Our bodies receive both internal and external cues to help keep us on track. Internal cues come from a brain structure called the *super chiasmatic nucleus* (SCN). This is the body clock, responsible for helping regulate sleep. We also receive external cues like exposure to light, the regularity of mealtimes, and exercise, which keep the body clock in sync with our environment. When we become out of sync with our biological clock, sleep problems can result. Working with our biological clock can increase sleep continuity and quality—and reduce nightmares.

Stages of Sleep

There are two main types of sleep: *rapid eye movement* (REM) sleep, and *non-rapid eye movement* (non-REM) sleep. Sleep is divided into four stages. We move through each of these stages roughly every ninety minutes to two hours. Healthy sleepers move through four to six of those cycles every night. The following chart breaks down the different sleep stages, though the time spent in each cycle changes some throughout the night.

Sleep Stage	Time Spent (percentage of sleep)	REM or Non-REM Sleep	Type	Dreams or Nightmares?
N1	1 to 5 minutes (5 percent)	Non-REM sleep	Light sleep, transitioning between wakefulness and sleep	Dreams can occur
N2	10 to 60 minutes (50 percent)	Non-REM sleep	Changes in brain activity with slower theta waves	Dreams can occur
N3	20 to 40 minutes (20 percent)	Non-REM sleep	Deepest sleep	Dreams can occur
REM	10 to 60 minutes (25 percent)	REM sleep	Paradoxical active memory consolidation	Nightmares most often occur

As you can see, dreams can occur in stages N1, N2, and N3, but they tend to be less vivid and more "thought like." These dreams may involve thinking about a problem or an experience but not have vivid images or a detailed storyline.

REM sleep is the stage where your nightmares are likely occurring. REM sleep is a more active stage of sleep. Sometimes people call this *paradoxical sleep*, because brain activity looks more like activity we have while awake. It has distinct biological features, like the type of brainwaves produced and the characteristic eye movements. The term "rapid eye movement" comes from the distinct way our eyes move rapidly behind our eyelids during sleep. Our bodies are doing a lot of important functions—including storing memories—during REM sleep. If you are experiencing nightmares, your REM sleep is likely disrupted. This may explain some common problems your nightmares may be causing, including difficulty with fatigue, mood, thinking, or behavior during the day.

Sleep Problems That Accompany Nightmares

When nightmares are occurring, we often see additional sleep struggles that might co-occur alongside, cause, or exacerbate the nightmares. They include the following sleep problems.

Insomnia Disorder

Nightmares and insomnia are frequently diagnosed in the same person. Insomnia is a condition in which people have difficulty falling asleep, staying asleep, or waking too early. If you struggle with one of these issues for thirty minutes or more, on three or more nights per week, you may have insomnia. While most people can think of a time when they've had trouble sleeping on an isolated occasion, insomnia disorder is diagnosed when this is a persistent problem (two weeks or more of constant sleep problems). Many of the skills used in this book to address nightmares will also help with your insomnia symptoms.

Obstructive Sleep Apnea

Some additional sleep problems need evaluation and treatment by a sleep physician. One common sleep problem that can occur with nightmares is *obstructive sleep apnea*, where people stop breathing many, many times in the night. Sleep is frequently disrupted because their body is trying to wake them up so they can resume breathing! How do you know if you may have obstructive sleep apnea? Some common symptoms are having a bed partner say you snore loudly or stop breathing while you sleep, having to use the restroom multiple times per night, waking with a headache, and profound sleepiness during the day even when you have gotten enough sleep. If you are encountering these issues, consider further assessment. Some wearable devices such as Apple Watches now claim to detect sleep apnea. Speak with your physician if you experience any symptoms.

Non-REM Parasomnias

Behaviors called *parasomnias* occur during non-REM sleep, and include things like sleep walking, sleep talking, and eating in your sleep. During these periods of time, people remain asleep but can appear awake. They may scream, move around, appear frightened, sweat, and be inconsolable. Sleep terrors or "night terrors," which we mentioned earlier, are sometimes confused with nightmares. But they actually fall into the group of non-REM parasomnias. During a sleep terror, it is difficult to awaken someone and they usually do not recall the experience. Sleep terrors are not dangerous, but they can be really distressing for others in the household. They are disorders of arousal that usually occur in N3 sleep, the deepest stage of sleep. They can occur in up to 40 percent of children and usually disappear by the teenage years, although some adults still experience night terrors.

Non-Nightmare REM Parasomnias

Some people experience REM sleep parasomnias other than nightmares. This REM sleep behavior disorder involves acting out a dream physically. This disorder is often associated with neurological disorders like Parkinson's disease. To be clear: some individuals with nightmares also act out their dreams (yelling, punching, kicking, for example), but REM sleep behavior disorder involves acting out nearly every dream and a great deal more movement. It is far less common than nightmare disorder. If you experience a lot of movement with your dreams, especially if you or anyone in your family have a history of Parkinson's disease, it's important to have this evaluated by a sleep physician. During REM, our body is designed to paralyze our big muscle groups to protect us from acting out our dreams, hurting ourselves, or our bed partners. In REM sleep behavior disorder, that mechanism can be broken so that people can have movements during sleep. It's also possible to awaken from sleep and feel paralyzed, unable to move voluntarily. This is called sleep paralysis. Sleep paralysis is usually harmless if it occurs once in a blue moon, but still scary! If it happens frequently, it can be a sign of potential narcolepsy. If you are noticing any of these problems in addition to nightmares, we strongly recommend you talk to a sleep physician.

Key Components of Nightmares

You can likely tell us a lot about your nightmares. Let's clearly define a nightmare disorder, before we move forward. There are multiple sets of criteria that can be used to define nightmares, but the key components are: content, distress, and wakening.

> **Content:** Nightmares are vivid, disturbing, or frightening dreams. They can contain content that is familiar, replicates a previous negative life event, or seems to appear randomly.

> **Distress:** Nightmares are upsetting, and many people experience bodily sensations such as a racing heart, shortness of breath, and fear.

> **Wakening:** Nightmares cause you to awaken, disrupting the sleep cycle. Immediately following a nightmare, you are usually awake and alert. The distressed bodily sensations many people experience are counter to the body state we need to return to sleep. Therefore, you likely have difficulty returning to sleep.

Nightmares typically occur during REM sleep and are more common during the second half of the night. You may also experience a dysphoric sensation, with difficulty distinguishing the waking world from your nightmare. It may take several minutes to transition from this sensation. Due to this sense of fear, you may purposefully stay awake or develop specific thoughts about what might happen if you return to sleep. For example: *I will have the nightmare again. I will die in my dreams and in real life.* If you have disturbing dreams that do not lead to awakenings or you cannot recall the content, that might be a different sleep problem. Some of the skills in this book may help with your symptoms, but we also recommend seeking out an evaluation with a trained sleep provider.

If you are having one nightmare per week, or more, it is likely distressing and impairing, and therefore important to treat. Ultimately, if nightmares disturb your sleep—regardless of frequency—the skills in the book will be helpful.

Why Do We Have Nightmares?

Scientists have developed several theories about why nightmares may occur, but there is no universal consensus. Let's look at some of these theories. See which one makes the most sense to you.

Trauma

Nightmares may be the brain's effort to make sense of difficult life experiences. That might make you think about trauma. Many people who've experienced trauma also experience nightmares. In fact, nightmares are a key symptom of PTSD. However, nightmares are not always trauma related.

Processing Experiences

Non-trauma nightmares are sometimes referred to as *idiopathic*. For instance, you may experience nightmares in response to periods of high stress or with strong negative emotions. To process those experiences, your brain works during REM sleep to consolidate and store those experiences. Key brain structures involved in REM sleep help us regulate our emotions. In fact, some scientists have proposed a biological model of nightmares called the *neurocognitive model of disturbing dreaming*. This model describes the efforts of several brain structures to process distress, fearful memories, or other negative events. When these systems successfully process strong emotions, the nightmares often resolve.

A Learned Behavior

Nightmares sometimes persist for months, years, or even decades. We have worked with Vietnam Era veterans in the United States who struggled with nightmares for forty-five or fifty years before receiving treatment. Nightmares as a learned behavior is commonly called a *cognitive behavioral* view of nightmares. In this view, the thoughts you have (cognitive) and behaviors that you engage in, as well as your emotions, can be possible causes of nightmares. They can also signal places for intervention.

Picture this. You have a poor night's sleep and then start to have some automatic thoughts about your sleep (or lack of sleep). If nightmares were the main cause, you might think about what it means to have nightmares, or how the nightmares will last forever. None of these thoughts are sleep promoting, they are more distress and wakefulness promoting.

Likewise, we can develop behaviors that lead to increased nightmares. You've likely never thought of it this way, but waking up from a dream is a behavior. It can be shaped like any other behavior. Waking up is one way we can escape or avoid nightmares. However, these awakenings are the very reason that we remember having the nightmare, and they disturb our sleep. So while wakeups help avoid the nightmare, they can have notable negative impacts on us and our sleep. The pattern becomes:

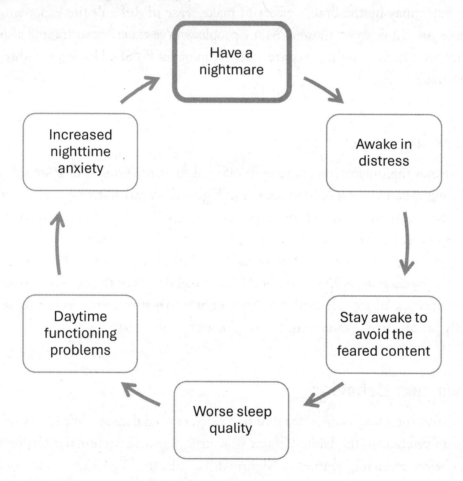

Then the cycle repeats. Moreover, we know that disrupted sleep one night can make nightmares more likely the next night. Escaping and avoiding nightmares is a short-term solution. The avoidance of nightmares increases sleep fragmentation, making you more likely to remember your dreams and perpetuating the nightmare problem. It's also possible that avoiding the nightmare may prevent exposure to the nightmare. While that may be your initial goal, continued avoidance sustains the nightmares. It prevents you and your brain from processing the content and emotions.

In this workbook, we apply this cognitive behavioral theory of nightmares to provide you with skills to break this cycle and experience relief from nightmares. There are also a host of materials available online, including additional support for children and trauma survivors, at https://www.newharbinger.com/55817. It is never too early, and it is never too late. Let's get started.

CHAPTER 2

Measure Sleep and Nightmares to Track Progress

As we start this journey of improving your sleep and nightmares, we want to explore what your sleep looks like right now. You will use the skills in this chapter to help measure progress across this program. You are likely good at knowing if you didn't sleep well. However, this can be hard to quantify without help. We want to give you a tool to measure your sleep (or lack of sleep) and nightmares. This will allow you to look for improvements as you use the skills in this book. Tracking your sleep and nightmares can help you celebrate small gains, know which skills are helpful, and know when you might need to try a different strategy.

Consider when you go to your primary care doctor. If your blood pressure is high, your doctor may recommend trying to reduce it through diet and exercise. If these efforts are unsuccessful, based on the next measurements, medication might be recommended. Another set of measurements would be taken after a trial of medication to assess response to treatment, and so on. In the same way, we hope you will measure your sleep and nightmares in order to decide if the skills you try are working for you.

My Current Sleep

There are a lot of ways we can measure sleep and nightmares. We will share how you can track your sleep shortly. Let's start with a few key areas that are often the top concerns of our patients. Which of the following are true for you? (Circle all that apply.)

General Sleep Problems

It's hard to fall asleep.	I wake up too much.	I sleep at the wrong times (falling asleep in the day).
I don't sleep enough.	I wake up too early.	My sleep is broken (not continuous).
I sleep too much during the day.	I avoid sleeping at night.	My sleep disrupts my loved ones.

Nightmares

My nightmares happen often and cause distress.

I can't function the next day because of my nightmares.

I am afraid to go to sleep because of nightmares.

I worry I will have more nightmares.

I cannot return to sleep if I have a nightmare.

My nightmares impact my relationships.

If I go back to sleep after a nightmare, I'm going to have the nightmare again.

Now pause for a moment. Think about what you would like your sleep to look like. Check all that apply.

I want my sleep to:

- ☐ Be more restful.
- ☐ Have fewer wake-ups!
- ☐ Have fewer nightmares!
- ☐ Be longer (with more hours).
- ☐ Be more consolidated at night (take fewer naps).
- ☐ _____
- ☐ _____
- ☐ _____

Many people set specific goals for how much time they want to sleep. You may have a goal of how long you want to sleep, but we encourage you to think about sleep quality and continuity.

Sleep quality is often about how refreshed you feel approximately fifteen to thirty minutes after awakening, as well as how you feel throughout the day. It's likely important to you to feel refreshed when you wake up—like you've had restorative sleep. So consider setting some goals based on how you are feeling and if you have the energy to perform tasks needed the next day. You might also set goals around how you want to feel around loved ones (for example, less irritable, more energy to play with your kids).

Sleep continuity is about sleeping in (mostly) one continuous block, and doing so leads to better daytime functioning. Many people with nightmares can sleep one to two complete sleep cycles (each sleep cycle is ninety minutes to two hours) before waking up from a nightmare. Do you notice a pattern in the timing of your nightmares? Maybe three to four hours after you fall asleep?

Take a few minutes to make some notes here about your sleep goals.

_____

_____

_____

_____

_____

_____

Tracking Your Sleep

One of the first tools we want to share with you is the sleep diary. This is how you will track your sleep during this program. First look at this sleep diary.

MEASURE SLEEP AND NIGHTMARES TO TRACK PROGRESS

Today's Date	**Sample:** Sunday, April 5th		
What time did you get into bed?	10:15 p.m.		
What time did you try to go to sleep?	11:30 p.m.		
How long did it take you to fall asleep?	55 minutes		
How many times did you wake up, not counting your final awakening?	3 times		
In total, how long did these awakenings last?	1 hour, 10 minutes		
What time was your final awakening?	6:35 a.m.		
What time did you get out of bed for the day?	7:20 a.m.		
How would you rate the quality of your sleep?	☐ Very poor ☒ Poor ☐ Fair ☐ Good ☐ Very good	☐ Very poor ☐ Poor ☐ Fair ☐ Good ☐ Very good	☐ Very poor ☐ Poor ☐ Fair ☐ Good ☐ Very good
Comments	I have a cold.		

Look at the example column in gray. Based on this limited information, there are a few areas this person may want to change.

1. **Time to fall asleep.** Around twenty minutes is the average amount for healthy sleepers to fall asleep. Bringing down this amount of time, lying in bed awake, could help this person's sleep overall.

2. **Nighttime awakenings.** Nighttime awakenings can be nightmare-related or not. Using the skills in this book can help with both types of awakenings.

3. **Early morning awakenings.** Some people wake up several hours before their desired wake time and have difficulty returning to sleep or may be unable to return to sleep. Staying in bed when this happens can increase symptoms of insomnia.

As you track your sleep for the next week or two, look for patterns in your sleep. Some people find it helpful to track the regularity of other things in their day like meals, exercise, light exposure, and medication. You can create extra spaces to add in these elements.

While considering your goals for this workbook, remember that you have choices about how you move forward. We would not recommend making all the possible changes at once! It's important to prioritize the parts of your sleep that you are willing to start working on now.

This diary tracks a few different elements of sleep. All these elements provide information about your sleep habits. They also present opportunities to use the skills in this book to target what's most important to you. For example:

- If you notice it takes a long time to fall asleep, you may want to try skills around relaxation (chapter 6) or stimulus control (chapter 9).

- If you're waking up in the middle of the night, are all those wake-ups due to nightmares? The skills in chapters 7 and 8, related to visualization and rescription, will help.

You can download a copy of the sleep diary by visiting https://www.newharbinger.com/55817. We recommend you complete a sleep diary each week you are working on this program. Improving your sleep can help improve your nightmares. You can also track these in a mobile app, and some apps will graph changes in your sleep for you. We recommend the free mobile app "Insomnia Coach" from the Department of Veterans Affairs. It also has a program for treating insomnia. Some of the tools we have in this workbook will overlap, but this workbook contains specific tools for nightmares that other resources do not.

The most important thing for now is to track what is happening in your sleep and look for patterns. Here are important rules about using a sleep diary:

- Always fill them out the next day.

- No clock watching! We are asking you to think about best estimates. Watching the clock often makes sleep problems worse.

- Look for patterns over time. We recommend at least five days of tracking, and you'll see patterns appearing better after about two weeks.

- There's also a space for comments on sleep diaries because sometimes a night of sleep does not reflect what is typical. Sometimes things happen in our lives that explain a bad night's sleep, other than sleep problems. These could be things like being sick, having bad weather in the area, or having to wake up to care for a family member. We encourage you to document those as well.

Tracking Your Nightmares

In this section, we also encourage you to track your nightmares. This part will be especially important as you look for changes in nightmare intensity, frequency, and the amount of control you feel over your nightmares. Here is an example of a nightmare diary.

THE NIGHTMARE & SLEEP DISORDER TOOLKIT

Today's Date	**Sample:** Sunday, April 5th		
At bedtime, my anxiety was a ____. (0 = no anxiety; 10 = worst anxiety)	3		
Last night, I had ____ number of nightmares.	2		
My nightmare severity was ____. (0 = not severe; 10 = extremely severe)	5		
I had ____ control over my nightmares. (0 = no control; 10 = complete control)	0		
Last night, I had ____ number of dreams.	0		
My emotions in my dream were ____. (0 = positive; 10 = negative)	0		
Last night I took or used _____ to help me sleep.	Sound machine		

This nightmare log has questions about how you felt going to sleep (anxiety rating), the number of nightmares, the severity of the nightmare, and how much control you had. We use severity ratings of 0 to 10 for these rating scales, with 5 as the midpoint.

For bedtime anxiety: A rating of 0 says you are calm and relaxed getting into bed. A 10 says you felt so anxious it was likely hard to be still and very difficult to fall asleep.

For nightmare severity: A rating of 0 means the nightmare was not disturbing. It probably was not even a nightmare! In contrast, a rating of 10 is the most disturbing, upsetting nightmare you could have; it probably was vivid in detail and you had some physical reactions. You really felt it in your body when you woke up. You may have strong emotional reactions even after you wake.

Control: This is something people find harder to rate. A rating of 0 would indicate you had no control over the nightmare or its content. A 10 means you had complete control of your nightmare.

Dreams: We include measures of dreams here as well. A lot of people do not recall dreams if they are pleasant, or do not recall them in the same detail as nightmares. As we work on reducing your nightmares, you may notice the number of dreams increases. Or you may not notice any change. If you do have dreams, we encourage you to rate the emotions in those dreams on a scale where 0 includes positive emotions, 5 is neutral, and 10 would be negative emotions.

Ongoing Sleep and Nightmare Tracking

As you continue to track your sleep and nightmares, come back to these next few sections often to review progress and receive some recommendations. As much as possible, we try to make these recommendations based on your own data to ensure your treatment is a good fit for you. After your first week (or two) of tracking, take a few minutes to reflect on your sleep and nightmare logs.

Do you see any patterns in your sleep logs for your bedtime and wake time? For example, if you go to bed later, does it take as long to fall asleep? Write about any differences in your nightmare frequency based upon your bedtime or wake time.

_____
_____
_____
_____

For some, tracking their sleep and nightmares can be impactful! You may confirm things like: you are having nightmares frequently, sleeping less than you thought, it is taking longer to fall asleep than you expected, or you have a lot of variability in your sleep from day to day or weeknights to weekends. You are not alone! When people are struggling with nightmares, their sleep patterns often become quite disrupted. Let's look at common reasons why.

Assessing Bedtimes and Wake Times

Does your log show you are staying in bed longer than you are sleeping or trying to "catch up" on sleep? This may cause more problems. You may say to yourself: *If I stay in bed longer (even if I'm not sleeping), I'm still getting rest!* Staying in bed longer backfires on a lot of patients with nightmares and insomnia. The more time you spend in bed awake, the more your body learns to be awake in bed.

Look at your sleep log, specifically at your bedtime and wake time. Across the first week, does your bedtime vary more than one hour per night? (It's normal to have some variability.)

What are the patterns for your bedtime and wake time?

- My earliest bedtime this week was: _____
- My latest bedtime this week was: _____

- The difference between these two times was: _____ minutes / hours (Circle one.)

Now let's look at wake time.

- My earliest wake time was: _____
- My latest wake time was: _____
- The difference between these two times was: _____ minutes / hours (Circle one.)

Variability in your bedtime and wake time can impact your sleep and nightmares in a few ways. For instance, while unexpected, you might have more nightmares on nights you sleep less (and not just because nightmares may make it difficult to fall back asleep). When we are in sleep debt, or we go to bed later than normal, we increase the proportion of REM sleep and increase the chances of having nightmares.

The wake time is most important when it comes to setting your circadian clock (more on that in a few chapters). For the next few weeks, we encourage you to consider setting a fixed wakeup time. Yes, even on weekends. We will also ask you to set an earliest bedtime—the earliest you would want to go to sleep. However, if you are not sleepy at that bedtime, stay up a little longer until you truly feel sleepy. This can help your body associate being in bed with being asleep.

Assessing Nightmares

Now let us turn to your nightmares log. Answer the following questions.

- This week I had _____ nightmares.
- My nightmares ranged in intensity from _____ to _____ (1 to 10 scale).
- Calculate an average by adding the ratings and dividing that total by the number of nightmares. My average nightmare intensity range was _____.

Are there variations in intensity from night to night? If so, this week you may want to pay closer attention to any things that influence your nightmares. The emotions you experience close to bedtime can set the tone for your nighttime emotions. Going to bed angry, irritated, or just amped up can make it more likely that you will have a nightmare. You may want to save watching that exciting show for another time.

You also might be fearful of having another nightmare. Fear of going to sleep, having a nightmare, or disturbances in your sleep environment can also affect your ability to fall asleep and increase the likelihood of nightmares.

Consider any factors that may have influenced your nightmares this week. Write them down.

_____

_____

_____

_____

_____

Patterns in your sleep can affect your nightmares. Are you having more nightmares after a good night of sleep? Or after a bad night of sleep? For most people, having a bad night of sleep leads to more distress in the daytime, more anxiety at bedtime, and worse sleep the next night—including more nightmares. You can start to disrupt this cycle by improving your sleep overall (chapter 5 will be especially helpful) and then move on to other skills to address nightmares.

Noticing Changes in Your Logs

Depending on how many days or weeks have passed since you started tracking, you may see different amounts of change. Changing sleep habits often takes time, but in the early stages you may see small changes that will add up over time. (If you are using a mobile app or other tool that calculates the time in bed, number of wake-ups, or sleep efficiency, consider that here too.) Considering the goals you set, continue to check in and answer the following questions. What changes are you seeing in the logs?

Are you being consistent with bedtime, wake time? **Yes   No**   (Circle one.)

Have you noticed decreases in nighttime anxiety? **Yes   No**   (Circle one.)

Have there been any changes in the frequency of your nightmares? **Yes   No**   (Circle one.)

Have there been any changes in the intensity of your nightmares? **Yes   No**   (Circle one.)

Have there been any changes in the level of control in your nightmares? **Yes   No**   (Circle one.)

Write down anything else that you want to check your logs going forward.

_____ **Yes   No**   (Circle one.)

_____ **Yes   No**   (Circle one.)

_____ **Yes   No**   (Circle one.)

Keep Tracking Sleep and Nightmares

While we can be aware that we are struggling with sleep, over time it can be difficult to recall how bad things were or to notice small incremental changes. Now that you know where you are starting from, continued tracking can help you measure progress. Tracking your sleep and nightmares ongoing will help you see those changes and know when you need to add in the next element to continue building your recovery. It may take a few weeks to see changes. If you are not seeing changes yet, it just means you need more practice.

It is important to use the sleep diary and nightmare tracking to measure progress! Sometimes it is not immediately clear what improvements we are making just from our subjective experience, but having the data in the sleep diaries helps illustrate what is improving, and where there is more work to be done. Sometimes the people around us can see changes before we can. Consider letting loved ones know you're working on your sleep. Check in with them about any progress they see over time. If you're using this workbook with a healthcare provider, let them know about your progress and share any successes or challenges.

We will ask you to reflect on how your sleep and nightmares have changed after you practice each element as you implement the sleep and nightmare recovery plan. In the next chapter, you'll consider the different treatment pathways available to you as you create that plan.

CHAPTER 3

Treatment Elements and Methods for Nightmares

There are many paths to better sleep, and there can be several "right" paths. In this chapter, you will learn about some of these paths and select the one you would like to take first. Each path is an evidence-based strategy for improving sleep in nightmare sufferers. They can come together to form a journey based on your individual goals and needs. Several of the elements we'll share can be helpful for anyone.

Treatment Skills You May Want to Learn

With many techniques and treatments for nightmares, clinicians usually do not use every tool for every patient; rather, they choose the ones that will likely work best for the patient. This makes sense, because everyone's situation is different. You'll use this "cafeteria approach" to tailor a treatment plan to your specific needs. Here is a brief description of each skill so you can decide which are best for you! You'll learn about them in depth in chapters to come.

Sleep Hygiene

Sleep hygiene is a well-known treatment for sleep. It often involves a sheet of behavioral dos and don'ts about factors like caffeine intake, bedroom temperature, and exercise habits. You might look over the list, choose a few behaviors you are willing to try (perhaps lowering the thermostat a bit at night) and reject those you are unwilling to do (such as reducing caffeine intake). But many people set the sheet aside and do not think about it again. This is unfortunate, because sleep hygiene behaviors can be very useful when followed. But many people discount its effectiveness because they don't understand the reasoning behind each suggestion. This is why, in the sleep hygiene section, we will help you understand why each recommendation is important for improving your sleep and reducing nightmares.

Have you tried sleep hygiene before? **Yes   No**   (Circle one.)

List the tips that you actually followed.

- _____
- _____

- _____
- _____

Why did you choose not to follow the others?

_____

_____

_____

Do you think you might try a few more behavior recommen-   **Yes   No**   (Circle one.)
dations if you understand how they can help?

Write down any aspects of incorporating sleep hygiene into your treatment plan that make you nervous or unsure.

_____

_____

_____

_____

Sleep Restriction

Despite its confusing—and perhaps alarming—name, sleep restriction is best thought of as fitting the right amount of sleep into one sleep period. There is only so much sleep your body can generate no matter how hard you try—for most it is six to eight hours. For those who have sleep problems, they will often spend ten to twelve hours in bed just to get that same six to eight hours of sleep! With sleep restriction, you figure out how much sleep you can generate and then create a sleep schedule that ensures you are actually asleep when you are in bed!

On average, how long do you typically spend in bed? How much sleep actually results?

_____
_____
_____

Stimulus Control

Similarly to how we can pair the sofa with snacks if we regularly snack while watching TV, you might associate your bed with being awake instead of being asleep. Stimulus control is a strategy that looks at all your cues for being asleep or awake. You want your body and brain to recognize that the bed is a place for sleep. If you've struggled with nightmares or insomnia, the bed often takes on additional meaning. Stimulus control works to pair the bed with sleep again, rather than nightmares, by only being in bed when you're asleep.

Do you often lie in bed for long periods without being able to sleep?   **Yes   No**   (Circle one.)

When your head hits the pillow, do you feel wide awake even if you felt sleepy beforehand?   **Yes   No**   (Circle one.)

Relaxation

Do you tend to feel anxious throughout the day and have trouble winding down? Do you worry or ruminate in bed? If so, relaxation can help you realize when you are holding stress and tension. We will teach you strategies to address this stress and increase relaxation. You can do them at home and on the go!

Visualization

Visualization is a relaxation strategy in which you create a detailed mental picture with sight, sounds, smells, thoughts, and feelings. Focusing on that mental picture can help you relax. Visualization is a vital part of most nightmare treatments that involve rescription, which we discuss next. This chapter will help you best visualize information to make it as vivid as possible and troubleshoot the challenges you may experience.

Rescription

Rescription is a core skill in nightmare treatment. It helps you take your existing nightmare story and rewrite it in a purposeful way, so you can choose what you dream about. It takes some practice during the day. Rehearsing and picturing the new story retrains the brain so it has a new pathway to replace the nightmares with a new dream. Rescription is very effective, with anecdotal reports of around 80 percent success rates. It can also be quite fun, as it will teach you how to make a nightmare into a dream you would really like to have. Although not everyone reports having the new dream, some do, and it can be a very exciting outcome.

If you could select your dreams and dream about anything you want, what would you pick?

_____

_____

_____

_____

Exposure

For those who need this skill, it is an absolute game changer! As you learn how to expose yourself to content you find frightening or anxiety-provoking, your anxiety can lessen. It's commonly (though not always) required for nightmares about trauma. But it's less needed for nightmares you have had from childhood without a trauma link. Exposure works by dulling those negative memories and images so they are not as disturbing as they used to be. So, do you need exposure? Our advice is to try imagery rescription first. Then, if you are still struggling with nightmares, we strongly encourage trying exposure. If you are uncertain, we give more details and examples in chapter 8.

Like sleep restriction, exposure is not the most pleasant activity. But the benefits can far outweigh the challenges. Would you be willing to actively engage with your nightmares, trying to vividly experience them until your anxiety decreased, in order to dull them going forward? Why or why not? What worries you about practicing exposure?

_____

_____

_____

_____

_____

Cognitive Restructuring

Do you struggle to go to sleep, or return to sleep if you wake up in the middle of the night, because of your thoughts? Do you battle worries all night and ruminate on things that keep you awake? If so, this is the tool for you! In the cognitive restructuring chapter, you will learn cognitive behavioral strategies. These skills can help reduce the amount of worry and rumination you have at night to help you sleep better. If you don't have problems with worry or rumination at night, then this is a topic you can safely skip.

Lucid Dreaming and Lucidity Checks

Lucid dreaming therapy teaches you strategies to become aware that you are asleep while you are having a dream so you can change the dream right when you are having it. For some people, lucid dreaming comes naturally, but for others it is a skill to learn. We will teach you about lucidity checks: activities you can do throughout the day to help determine if you are awake or asleep. The more you do this during the day, the more you will do it while asleep. This helps you determine when you are asleep in a dream, so you can take control! We view lucid dreaming as a third-choice treatment and recommend trying rescripting and exposure first. But if you want to take the wheel of your dreams, or prefer this strategy, go ahead and read this chapter.

If you would like to learn to become aware of when you are asleep, so you can take control of your dreams, what would you like to do in that dream?

_____

_____

_____

_____

_____

_____

Treatment Methodologies for Nightmares

Now you know the skills involved. Next, we'll show you how formal nightmare treatment therapies use them differently. You do not have to select one treatment or another. Instead, you can take some pieces from one or more of the interventions and add other pieces. In the next chapter, you'll use them to create the treatment path that's best for you and your goals.

Imagery Rehearsal Therapy

Imagery rehearsal therapy (IRT) is the nightmare intervention with the most empirical support. You learn how to change your nightmare into a dream you would like to have (rescription) and practice it using visualization. IRT can include sleep hygiene and stimulus control, especially if you are also struggling with insomnia. IRT with exposure can be especially helpful for trauma-related nightmares, or if you only partially respond to rescription.

Key elements of IRT include:

- Visualization
- Rescription
- Sleep hygiene (optional)
- Exposure (optional)

IRT might be effective:

- When you have trauma and non-trauma nightmares.
- For all ages, including kids, with modifications such as drawing a rescripted dream.

IRT might *not* be effective when:

- Your dreams are a direct replay of a trauma, but it is still likely worth trying first.

Do you like the idea of being able to change your dream? Why or why not?

_____

_____

_____

_____

_____

_____

Does this feel like an easy intervention for you, or one you may struggle with? Why or why not?

_____

_____

_____

_____

_____

Cognitive Behavioral Therapy for Insomnia

When your sleep is improved, you usually have fewer nightmares. Or you are less likely to be awakened by your nightmares, which can be an improvement since you typically won't remember a dream if you don't wake up during it. Cognitive behavioral therapy for insomnia (CBT-I) focuses on improving quality of sleep. It's primarily for individuals with insomnia, but it may also benefit nightmare sufferers.

Key elements of CBT-I include:

- Sleep hygiene (optional)
- Stimulus control
- Sleep restriction
- Cognitive restructuring

CBT-I might be effective when:

- You have difficulty going to sleep, staying asleep, waking up too early—or any combination of these problems.

CBT-I might *not* be effective when:

- There is a history of bipolar disorder or you have limited mobility; in these cases, you should work with a professional and omit elements like sleep restriction.

Exposure, Relaxation, and Restriction Therapy

As you can see by its name, exposure, relaxation, and restriction therapy (ERRT) includes similar elements to CBT-I and IRT but adds therapeutic exposure and relaxation to the nightmare. It also builds on the original nightmare when rescripting a new dream. The treatment was created for those with trauma nightmares. But if you are not getting enough relief from IRT, the additional elements in ERRT may be helpful.

Key elements of ERRT include:

- Visualization
- Rescripting
- Exposure
- Relaxation
- Sleep hygiene (optional)

ERRT might be effective when:

- You have trauma nightmares and IRT alone is not sufficient to provide relief.

Lucid Dreaming

It is estimated that about 25 percent of people are lucid dreamers, meaning they're aware that they are dreaming and are able to take control of the dream. If this is you, or if you would like to learn how to change your dreams while having them, lucid dreaming may be the easiest path for treating your nightmares. This approach is similar to IRT and ERRT, but it changes the dream in a very different way. Rather than practice a new dream, lucid dreaming teaches you how to realize when you are having a nightmare *while having it* so you can change your dream while you sleep!

In the following chart, you can see how these elements of sleep treatments fit under each type of treatment. You will notice that there is some overlap.

	CBT-I	IRT	ERRT	Lucid Dreaming
Sleep hygiene	X	X	X	X
Sleep restriction	X			
Stimulus control	X		X	
Visualization	(optional)	X	X	
Exposure		(optional)	X	
Rescription		X	X	
Cognitive restructuring	X	(optional)	(optional)	
Lucidity checks				X
Relaxation	(optional)	X	X	

Now that we have introduced you to the elements that are common, we want to help you determine the path that makes the most sense for you. In the chapters to come, you're going to use these elements as a framework for thinking about the different ways you can achieve better quality sleep.

CHAPTER 4

Choosing a Path for Nightmare Recovery

As you choose your own elements of treatment for your nightmares, you'll need to collect data to guide your decisions. Despite there being packages of interventions, there really is not a one-size-fits-all solution, as different skills are important for different people. The most common and well-researched treatment for nightmare sufferers includes items from sleep hygiene, visualization, exposure, and rescription. In this chapter, we will build upon the last chapter by helping you individualize your own treatment.

With a lot of paths to take, we will offer signposts and choices to help you move through the different elements. Continue tracking how your sleeping and nightmares are changing across time so that you know what elements may be helpful for you. After each chapter, we'll offer recommendations for what you might need to do. But know that all these resources are available to you at any time. Consider what you've learned about the different elements so far and your preferences. For instance:

- Is insomnia a struggle? If so, try skills like sleep hygiene, sleep restriction, and stimulus control.

- Do you want to dip a toe in to see how a few skills help, before going further? Try visualization and rescription before adding other skills.

- Are you willing to put the work in, do not mind challenging skills, and want them all? All elements are viable paths, so to start, pick what you are most comfortable with.

Take a few minutes to review the skills and add your preferences to this chart by checking the boxes and recording your thoughts.

CHOOSING A PATH FOR NIGHTMARE RECOVERY

	Willing to try!	Not willing to try.	Unsure or need more information.	Reasons for this choice.
Sleep hygiene				
Sleep restriction				
Stimulus control				
Visualization				
Exposure				
Rescription				
Cognitive restructuring				
Lucidity checks				
Relaxation				

As we shared in chapter 3, some skills are harder than others. For instance, exposure therapy relies upon facing something that causes you anxiety or distress, whereas relaxation is typically quite easy and enjoyable. For each skill in the following table, we have assigned a difficulty rating to give you a sense of how challenging it is. Knowing this can help you determine which skills you want to build into your plan and what order you want to follow as you tackle them.

Skills	Difficulty Level (1 = easiest; 5 = hardest)
Sleep hygiene and relaxation	2 for sleep hygiene, 1 for relaxation
Visualization	2
Rescription (after visualization)	2
Sleep restriction and stimulus control	4 for sleep restriction, 3 for stimulus control
Lucidity checks	3
Cognitive restructuring	4

Now it's time to explore creating a sleep and nightmare recovery plan. We like to think about the recovery plan as a living document. You can consistently edit and make changes throughout your recovery journey. The best plan uses all the evidence-based skills that you're willing to follow. So, for example, if you think sleep restriction sounds like a good idea, but it's not one you want to use or try, don't put it in your plan. To help you create your plan, here are three patients with different goals and needs to consider.

Making a Plan for John

John is a combat veteran who served two tours in Vietnam. He has been struggling with nightmares for nearly forty years now! John struggles with going to sleep and expects to have a nightmare every night. He tries splashing his face with cold water right before bed and sometimes tries to stay awake. Unfortunately, avoiding sleep has worsened John's nightmares. He wakes up with strong physical symptoms, like shortness of breath and a racing heart. Once awake, he gets up to check the doors and windows in his house, and then struggles to go back to sleep. During his nightmare, John feels out of control and it is very difficult to gain any type of control. He doesn't really think it's possible to get rid of the nightmares entirely.

John is reporting both insomnia and nightmares, so it makes sense to include skills from CBT-I, which is an insomnia treatment, in addition to nightmare interventions. Further, since John's nightmares are trauma-based, it may be necessary to include exposure to adequately address them.

John's Sleep Logs

John's first week of sleep tracking shows he may go to bed anytime between 9:45 p.m. and midnight. His wake time varies less, from 5:25 a.m. to 6:45 a.m., but some days he may remain in bed for a few more hours. He gets out of bed from fifteen minutes to almost two hours after waking up. This variability makes it difficult for John's body clock to keep a rhythm, and the extra time in bed trains his body that the bed does not always signal sleep. John's sleep log also shows there are large gaps when awake.

Paired with his nightmare log, John can see he's experiencing a lot of anxiety at bedtime, severe nightmares when he wakes, and often multiple nightmares in a night. The nightmares vary in severity, and he feels like he has no control. John's experience is similar to many patients we have treated over the years and gives us a lot of areas to work on with skills from this book. If you would like to review his logs, you can download them online at https://www.newharbinger.com/55817.

John's Goals

At this point in his recovery, John wants to sleep through the night and reduce the number or severity of trauma-related nightmares. To help him think about how he might measure progress, Johns filled out this chart.

Goal	What does that mean for you?	How will you measure progress?	Other notes
To sleep through the night.	I get about seven hours of sleep.	I will sleep from about midnight to 7 a.m.	
To reduce the number or severity of trauma-related nightmares.	I have fewer nightmares overall and fewer nights with nightmares. The nightmares aren't as severe.	I have nightmares fewer nights per week (three nights out of seven). When I do have a nightmare, the severity rating is less than 3.	I'm not sure I can have 0 nightmares ever, so I'll feel relieved if they ease up some.

John's goals don't include not having nightmares anymore. You may or may not have that goal. John wants to show a meaningful improvement in symptoms and to create a checkpoint to see how he is progressing and whether treatment needs to be altered. Once the goals recorded in the chart are met, he can make new goals to further reduce nightmares and sleep problems.

John's Final Plan

To improve John's sleep overall, he is going to start with sleep hygiene and relaxation. John has a lot of variability in his bedtime and wake time, and sleep hygiene will help him have more regular bedtimes and wake times. He reports a lot of nighttime anxiety, so he liked the idea of using some relaxation strategies both during the day and at bedtime.

Because John has trauma-related nightmares, he also wants to work on exposure and rescription. John's goals for exposure are to gain a greater feeling of control over the nightmare. He is not excited about approaching it, but he thinks looking at the nightmare more closely while awake can help him figure out how to rescript it. To help build up his skills for rescription, he is choosing to learn visualization skills beforehand. John is not sure he needs to work on his thoughts about his nightmares, so he wrote "maybe" for cognitive restructuring. John will continue tracking his sleep and nightmares to help to guide this path.

CHOOSING A PATH FOR NIGHTMARE RECOVERY

John has trouble with insomnia, but he's not sure if it's because of his nightmares or is a separate issue. Because of that, he has decided to add in stimulus control and sleep restriction—but has them set as a later skill, in case his insomnia is treated by addressing the nightmares. If it is not and he still struggles with insomnia once the nightmares improve, however, then he will begin working on these skills. Here is John's plan.

Order	Skills	Goal
1st	Sleep hygiene or relaxation	To help with sleeping through the night and reducing daytime anxiety.
2nd	Visualization	To help with relaxation and learning to do rescription.
3rd	Rescription	Change the content of nightmares into dreams I would like to have.
4th	Sleep restriction and stimulus control	Improve sleep to aid in sleeping through the night to address my insomnia.
5th	Exposure	Habituate to past trauma to reduce its negative effects.
Maybe?	Cognitive restructuring	Address negative thoughts that may be impacting my sleep.

There are many people who never served in the military or have another trauma that contributes to their nightmares. All kinds of people have nightmares, for varying reasons. So for another example, let's turn to Sarah.

Making a Plan for Sarah

Sarah is on the faculty of a large university, where she works as an assistant professor. Sarah has been having nightmares for a year now. These nightmares are not related to any particular trauma, but they create strong anxiety in the night. Sarah dreams there is someone else in her room, perhaps an intruder, and that she is in danger. These dreams cause her to startle awake. She spends a few minutes trying to figure out whether or not anyone is actually there. After going to the bathroom, splashing cold water on her face, and trying to relax in bed, Sarah can return to sleep. This happens several times each night.

Sarah's Sleep Logs

Sarah's log has good consistency overall for her bedtime and matches her report that she can fall asleep pretty quickly (fifteen minutes on average). She also has good consistency in her wake time, which means Sarah's circadian rhythm, or body clock, is working well. Her main complaint was about middle-of-the-night awakenings. She had awakenings on five nights—some of those were multiple times in a night, with up to an hour awake. This is disrupting her sleep, and she rates her sleep quality as poor. In her nightmares log, we can see she is anxious at bedtime, which may contribute to more nightmares. She also reports high nightmare severity ratings on the nights she has nightmares.

You can see Sarah's logs at https://www.newharbinger.com/55817.

Sarah's Goals

At this point in her recovery, Sarah's two main goals are to sleep through the night and to reduce the number or severity of nightmares.

Goal	What does that mean for you?	How will you measure progress?	Other notes
To sleep through the night.	I get about 7.5 hours of sleep.	I will sleep from about 10:30 p.m. to 6 a.m.	Have to get up at 6 a.m. to get everything done before my commute to work.
To reduce the number or severity of nightmares.	Not have as many nightmares, and they will be less intense or vivid.	Reduce bedtime anxiety to help reduce nightmares and the intensity. When I do, the intensity rating is 2 or less.	I need to reduce bedtime anxiety, and try to get it below a 4 rating.

Sarah's goals are very similar to John's. She doesn't expect to immediately stop having nightmares, as she recognizes that this is a skill that takes time to build. Rather, the initial goal is to show a meaningful improvement in these symptoms, and she'll form subsequent goals once she has met these.

Sarah's Final Plan

Sarah's situation does not seem to include insomnia as well as nightmares, and the nightmares are not trauma-related. Because of this, Sarah opts to not include the strategies from CBT-I (like sleep hygiene, stimulus control, sleep restriction) or exposure. However, she does decide she wants to include relaxation and visualization since her anxiety is high at bedtime, and she hopes reducing her anxiety will help reduce her nightmares. She could benefit from new dream content, so she plans to try rescription. Sarah's plan looks like this.

Order	Skills	Goal
1st	Relaxation	To reduce anxiety during the day and right before bed.
2nd	Visualization	To help with relaxation and learn to do rescription.
3rd	Rescription	To change the content of my nightmares into dreams I would like to have.

Although it is a basic plan, we have seen many nightmare sufferers recover fully with just these elements of treatment. However, should Sarah not get the results she desires after trying these three skills, she can always add more. Doing so depends on how she is feeling and what challenges she is facing at the end of treatment.

Let's look at one final example before you make your own plan. Toni is an example of someone who has experienced trauma but isn't sure if the trauma is influencing her nightmares.

Making a Plan for Toni

Toni is a nurse who was injured in a motor vehicle accident about five years ago and has been having nightmares ever since. Her nightmares have been increasing in frequency over the last six months with increased stress at work and increased caregiving needs for her aging parents. Toni is not sure if her nightmares are trauma related. They have a theme of helplessness, as in the dreams she's unable to take care of her patients and she doesn't know how to respond to medical emergencies. This was previously a strength of hers, given her long medical career. In life, Toni has started freezing during medical procedures. She has a lot of negative thoughts and guilt about this. The nightmares are the same, in that someone goes into cardiac arrest on her hospital floor, requiring emergency care. Who the patient is changes, sometimes even looking like family members or friends. Those dreams are especially upsetting, and Toni worries her loved ones may have a real medical emergency like the ones in her nightmares.

Toni's Sleep Log

In Toni's sleep log, there is a lot of variability in her sleep due to her sometimes having to do shift work, with her bedtime varying between 10:30 p.m. and 1:30 a.m. However, in part because she is so sleep deprived, she is able to fall asleep almost immediately and is even able to return to sleep after her nightmares. Yet the nightmares fragment her sleep, leading to one or more awakenings most nights. With the anxiety she has about having a nightmare, her sleep quality is poor.

She also finds that the nights she has nightmares correlates with significant anxiety the next day, and she has low mood. Unfortunately, having days like this makes it more likely that she will have a nightmare the next night, creating a negative cycle. In her treatment, along with getting some relief from her nightmares, she would love to get help with her anxiety. To see Toni's logs, visit https://www.newharbinger.com/55817.

Toni's Goals

At this point in her recovery, Toni has three main goals: to improve sleep quality by reducing nights with nightmares, to reduce the number or severity of nightmares, and to reduce the amount of nightmare anxiety and worry.

Goal	What does that mean for you?	How will you measure progress?	Other notes
To improve sleep quality.	To get more solid sleep; not stay awake worrying.	No more than one wake-up or when I wake up, I return to sleep within fifteen minutes.	
To reduce the number or severity of trauma-related nightmares.	I have fewer nightmares overall or fewer nights with nightmares or the nightmares aren't as severe.	I have nightmares fewer nights per week (three nights out of seven) or when I do, the severity rating is less than 3.	I'm not sure I can have 0 nightmares ever, I'll just take a reduction.
To reduce the anxiety and worry before bedtime.	Being able to rest and relax easier and aid in falling asleep.	50 percent reduction on how worried I feel before bed on a 1 to 10 scale.	

Toni's Final Plan

Since Toni reports significant anxiety, she is going to add both relaxation and cognitive therapy skills. She has a trauma history, but is not sure if the dreams are related to trauma or not. Toni is willing to do exposure but would like to use the other tools available before so she can hopefully avoid it. Because of this, she has added in lucidity checks for lucid dreaming in case she does not get enough relief from doing rescription. This gives her another intervention to try before she moves on to exposure. If after doing lucidity checks and lucid dreaming, she is still struggling with nightmares, she plans on trying exposure.

Order	Skills	Goal
1st	Relaxation	To reduce anxiety during the day and right before bed.
2nd	Visualization	To help with relaxation and learn to do rescription.
3rd	Rescription	To change the content of nightmares into dreams I would like to have.
4th	Cognitive therapy	To reduce anxiety during the day and right before bed.
If needed.	Lucidity checks and lucid dreaming	To learn to control dreams so I can change negative ones while having them.
If needed.	Exposure	To reduce the severity of nightmares and help me sleep through them.

Questions About Your Treatment Plan

Now it's time to consider what type of plan will best help you. There are some questions we commonly hear at this point, so we'll answer them in the hope that you gain even more clarity before you create your treatment plan.

Should I Include Insomnia Treatment?

It may or may not be obvious that you're experiencing insomnia and nightmares, or just nightmares. A good way to assess this is to look at your sleep log!

- Are you taking thirty minutes or more to fall asleep more than three times per week?
- What about waking up thirty minutes or more after you first fall asleep?
- Do you wake up without being able to fall back asleep?

If you experience these challenges regularly, especially if you are having them on nights that do not involve nightmares, then adding in the insomnia interventions (sleep restriction, stimulus control, sleep hygiene, cognitive therapy) might be a good idea.

Should I Include Exposure Therapy?

Believe it or not, this is one of the biggest debates in the nightmare field. Even the two authors of this workbook do not fully agree on when to use exposure. But we agree that if you have a trauma history, and your nightmares are about your trauma, it should be considered. Some nightmare clinicians believe it should be included regardless of trauma content. Others advocate that you do visualization and rehearsal first, see how much your sleep is improved, and then use exposure if you are still struggling.

Ultimately, this is your call. Which path feels better to you? *Include it* if you don't mind doing exposure to reduce the impact of your trauma or want a larger treatment dose from the beginning—adding relaxation, as they're commonly paired. *Don't include it* if exposure makes you nervous or you don't want to—perhaps trying visualization and rescription. Research shows that those with a trauma history can get significant relief from doing just rescription. If those skills do not resolve your nightmares, you could move on to include either to exposure or lucid dreaming. There are so many tools you can use!

Making Your Plan

Now that you've seen recovery plans for John, Sarah, and Toni, it's your turn! We'll guide you through the process of determining the right plan for you.

Choosing Goals

John and Sarah had common goals, as these goals fit the vast majority of nightmare sufferers seeking treatment. They are percentage-based and not dependent on hitting a firm number of nightmares per night. However, feel free to tweak them so they feel reasonable to you as guideposts for checking in and reassessing your progress. Your goals can (and will) be changed and modified as time goes on. You can also decide to include other goals, such as for insomnia. For example, you may want to reduce the number of nights per week that you are awake thirty minutes or more.

Write down at least two goals.

1. _____
_____

2. _____
_____

3. _____
_____

4. _____
_____

Now write those goals in the following chart. Consider how you define each of them and how you will measure progress.

CHOOSING A PATH FOR NIGHTMARE RECOVERY

Goal	What does that mean for you?	How will you measure progress?	Other notes

What skills are you planning to try? List them in the order you plan to do them. Then write down how the skills will help you reach your goals.

	Skills	Goal
1st		
2nd		
3rd		
4th		
5th		

Moving Between Skills

Since this is a skill-based intervention, it takes some time to learn and improve each skill before you have it mastered. Work on each skill for approximately a week before moving to the next skill. This gives you enough time to master the skill before moving to the next. You want slow, steady progress. Use your sleep and nightmare logs to monitor this progress. If you're unsure of progress from the logs, consider your daytime functioning. Do you feel rested within fifteen to thirty minutes of waking? Do you have more energy or willingness to engage in activities? Some signs of progress may include a few more "good nights" or feeling less anxious at bedtime. Whether you feel like you have mastered something, or you want more time to develop the skill, you can modify the amount of time you spend with each skill. For example, if you have done visualization in the past, you may find that you need less time with it. That said, practicing each skill for a week will keep you moving through the skills at a reasonable clip, with enough time and focus for you to master them. With your goals and treatment plan initiated, you are ready to turn to the chapter about the first skill you will use.

CHAPTER 5

Sleep Hygiene

If you've been struggling with your sleep, you have likely seen a list of recommendations from Internet searches, medical providers, or friends that are supposed to help you sleep. They include things like, "You should sleep in a cold, dark room" or "Don't drink too much caffeine." While these recommendations can be helpful, many times they're provided without clear explanations of how they connect to sleep and sleep cycles. As a result, many try these tools for a few days and do not see results. But they are an important part of a larger toolkit to address problematic sleep. Using them consistently is key. They also build a foundation for other sleep and nightmare interventions. It's true that not every skill works for every person.

In this chapter, we encourage you to personalize your plan, choosing to make the changes to meet your individual needs. We review evidence-based strategies with clear rationales for how they promote healthy sleep. This way, you'll be more likely to engage them consistently. It starts with understanding the basic daily routine of sleeping and waking.

The Sleep Wake Cycle

You may have heard of the *circadian rhythm*, which translates from Latin to mean "about a day." A day on Earth is roughly twenty-four hours long. Humans are designed to spend part of those hours asleep—usually the night, when it's dark. Sleep and wakefulness occur in this 24-hour cycle.

To improve sleep, you need to work with your body's circadian rhythm (also known as your "internal clock") to help bring your sleep back on track. In chapter 1, we described a part of your brain called the suprachiasmatic nucleus (SCN). This is the body clock that helps regulate your sleep and wake cycle, every 24 hours. Your brain receives signals from the environment, called *zeitgebers,* that help guide the circadian rhythm. For example, light helps tell your brain when it is daytime and nighttime. So it's helpful to get sunlight first thing in the morning and avoid blue light at night. In her work as a nurse, Toni notices that on days when she is exposed to the fluorescent lights at the hospital, especially later in her shifts, she has a harder time going to sleep at night. John has safety concerns, so he leaves lights on in his room all night. This might ease his anxiety, but it contributes to wakefulness. If you scroll your phone at night, you may have noticed that many phones and tablets now have a night mode that changes the light of your screen. The screen's emission of blue light signals your brain that it is daytime, so without night mode it can keep you awake. All this light gives conflicting signals to your circadian rhythm, as your brain looks for darkness as a cue for sleep and for timing of light during the day to help set your internal clock.

Think about your own experiences. When has light impacted your sleep? Was this a helpful or unhelpful experience?

_____

_____

_____

_____

_____

_____

Dreams and nightmares affect your sleep, likely impacting your sleep cycles at more time points than just waking up distressed. After nightmares, your sleep may be fragmented by the periods of wakefulness. If so, you may nap during the day to "catch up" on sleep. Sometimes it might feel safer to sleep during the day. Or you may sleep for shorter periods of time. In this way, nightmares may have pulled your sleep out of sync with your biological clock. They may force you into sleep deprivation and you are constantly trying to catch up.

Although taking a nap or sleeping in seemingly makes sense (to make up for loss of sleep), it commonly has the reverse effect and leads to further sleep problems! The reason why is the *homeostatic sleep drive*. Here's how it works. Think of your sleep drive like a gas tank. You hope to be all the way on empty when you go to bed. After "fueling up" all night as you sleep, you wake in the morning with a full tank. So when you either extend sleep (by sleeping in) or take naps during the day, not only are you not burning energy through activity, but you're putting more in the gas tank. As a result, you get to bedtime with a quarter tank of energy left. Some people are unable to fall asleep until they have burned this energy off. Others hit their tank's capacity too early in the night. Since they started sleeping with a quarter tank, they wake in the middle of the night or earlier than they would like.

While it might be hard, we recommend maintaining constant bed and wake times—as much as possible. Don't chase after lost sleep through sleeping in, taking naps, or going to bed early. They can all change your cycle and get your sleep off its rhythm. Instead, think this way: *If I don't get enough sleep tonight, I will sleep that much better tomorrow.* If you must nap, limit your sleep time to no more than thirty minutes. This is enough time to feel rejuvenated, but not so long that you drastically alter your homeostatic sleep drive. That said, if you can skip the nap, we strongly recommend it so your tank is empty at bedtime. Sometimes a short safety nap is needed (like before driving), especially for people with co-occurring sleep apnea or narcolepsy.

Improving Sleep Quality

Getting quality sleep can help reduce nightmares. There are a few key pieces to improving your sleep. Regular bed and wake times help to keep your body on track! Of these two, the wake time is the most important.

Why Keep a Consistent Wake Time? We recommend that you wake up at the same time every day, even on weekends! We know, it can be challenging to do this, but it will help improve your sleep and therefore your nightmares. Wake at the same time, whether you had a good night of sleep or a bad night of sleep. This regular wake time gives feedback to your body clock, the SCN, and helps your tank empty so you can begin building sleep drive for the next night.

Why Is a Regular Bedtime Important? You may be thinking, *Bedtime? But I'm an adult!* It can feel strange to set a bedtime for yourself. But when you're training your body clock, consistency and sleepiness must be your guide. For bedtime, you want to go to bed about the same time every night. Routines are key for sleep, as they can help prime the brain for sleep. So the more consistency around bedtime, including when that time is, the better. The exception is, you want to get into bed only when you are sleepy.

Distinguishing Sleepiness from Tiredness

Many people do not think much about the difference between being *sleepy* and being *tired*. This is an important distinction in sleep treatment. Here's an overview.

Sleepiness is:	Tiredness can be:
• A strong biological drive for sleep • A feeling of drowsiness that cannot be overcome easily • The sensations that your eyes are heavy and your head is drooping	• Physical (after a workout) • Emotional (after a difficult conversation) • Mental (after working on your taxes) • A combination of these things

Tiredness can usually be overcome by rest, engaging in a favorite activity, or with other supports. The next time you are tired, test this out by turning on your favorite song. You will likely feel more energetic, and the tiredness will lessen.

Sleepiness is different, as it is a biological drive. You cannot overcome sleepiness so easily. You may have experienced this when you watch a movie you really want to see, but no matter what you do, you keep dozing off and having to rewind. It happens while reading, when you close your eyes for just a moment but then realize you don't remember the last page. Sleepiness is the feeling you want when entering the bed. Of course, you can be BOTH sleepy and tired at the same time, but sleepiness should be your cue for going to bed.

So, if you set a bedtime of 11:00 p.m. but don't notice sleepiness, wait before getting into bed. Many people who struggle with sleep have difficulty tuning in to sensations of sleepiness. Over the next week, pay attention to when your body is giving you the following cues. Take some notes in your sleep diary.

- Are you noticing your eyelids getting heavy?
- Is it harder to pay attention to television, your book, or someone talking to you?
- Does your body feel relaxed and maybe heavy?

What else do you notice when sleepy?

_____

_____

_____

Your Bedtime and Wake Time Routine

Get your sleep diaries and look at them, keeping your routine in mind. Fill in the following worksheet.

My earliest bedtime this week was: _____

My latest bedtime this week was: _____

My earliest wake time this week was: _____

My latest wake time this week was: _____

Are your bedtimes and wake times regular (even on the weekend)?

Circle one: **They are routine (within thirty minutes to an hour).** **They vary.**

If you are already keeping regular bedtimes and wake times—great job! If you notice variations (yes, even on weekends), try working on this in the next week. How much do these times vary? What could you do this week to help make sleeping and waking more regular?

_____

_____

_____

_____

Control—Get Up and Out of Bed!

You can invite sleep by creating a relaxed environment. But you cannot control whether you sleep. For example, we advise waiting to go to bed until you are sleepy—even if it's past your scheduled bedtime. Getting into bed when you are not sleepy creates an association between your bed and being awake. We tend to pair objects together with enough repetition. For instance, if you always eat your favorite snack on the sofa, over enough pairings you'll sit down on the sofa and start craving that snack! Bed is the same way: you can pair being in your bed with being awake or being asleep.

It's surprisingly easy to pair bed with being awake. If you lie in bed trying to fall asleep or hoping to go back to sleep, you are pairing bed with being awake (and probably irritation), not being asleep! You may have this problem if:

- You feel very tired at home, but as soon as your head hits the pillow, you suddenly feel energized and wide awake.

- You use your bed for sleep, but also for working or studying, eating, watching television, or talking on the phone.

- You sleep better when traveling or in a hotel.

If any of these are true, you likely associate your bed with wakefulness instead of sleepiness. Think about college students in small dorm rooms. Their beds are for sleep, studying, gaming, hanging out with friends, and messaging. When they go to bed, their bodies and brains have a whole menu of activity choices. The same thing is true for people who struggle with sleep, as they spend more time in bed awake, trying to rest or fall asleep. This strategy makes sense, but it often backfires! Spending more time in bed usually does not result in more sleep. It usually results in more fragmented sleep with more periods of being awake.

Additionally, many people with nightmares have developed some negative associations with bed. *The bed is where I have nightmares, where I feel fearful and anxious.* This might lead you to sleep in places other than your bed and bedroom, which decreases the likelihood that you will sleep soundly in bed. If you are a trauma survivor who experienced the trauma at night or in a bed or bedroom, then you may also have associations with a darkened bedroom. This can cause even greater reactivity. Your body might start to have conditioned fight-or-flight reactions. This increased reactivity and distress make quality sleep less likely, and nightmares more likely. Nightmare sufferers are in a vicious cycle and don't know how to escape it. This is where *stimulus control* can help. In fact, it has some of the strongest evidence for effectiveness in helping improve sleep—of any sleep intervention! Due to association, we recommend setting two limits.

First, use your bed to sleep and for sexual activity only. Don't watch television, read, or have important conversations there. Get into bed only when you feel sleepy.

Second, once in bed, if you notice agitation or negative thoughts about sleep, do not remain in bed for more than fifteen minutes. Don't stare at the clock; just roughly estimate that fifteen minutes have passed. Then get out of bed, ideally move to another room, and do something that won't wake you too much but also that you enjoy (or at least do not mind). Blue light can wake you, so don't use a computer, smart phone or tablet. Watching television or reading a book printed on paper are both fine.

We know this can be difficult. When you have a bad night or a lot of nightmares, you may already be sleep deprived from all the awakenings! However, staying in bed awake gives your body feedback that staying awake in bed is okay, which only makes the problem worse. If you find you worry or are distressed in bed, it can also condition your body to respond this way at night.

Check all that apply. Do you:

☐ Lie in bed worrying about not sleeping?

☐ Tell yourself, *If I'm not sleeping, I'm at least resting?*

☐ Feel tired but wired at the same time? (We'll soon discuss nighttime anxiety.)

☐ Want to avoid bedtime, or the bed?

If you checked any of these boxes, you need to break these habits. Consider planning something enjoyable when you first wake up, such as setting the coffeemaker to start brewing before your alarm goes off. Having something to look forward to can help overcome that desire to stay in bed and help you stay true to your wake time.

Take a moment to think about something enjoyable you can do and write it down. Suggestions include calling a loved one, preparing a special breakfast, enjoying your morning beverage on the porch, stretching, or exercising.

_____

_____

_____

We suggest that as part of your morning routine, you push back the east-facing curtains, walk to the mailbox, or sit beside a window. Exposure to natural light, either in the morning or early afternoon (go outside at your lunch break), can help signal that you are awake for the day. It ensures that your circadian rhythm stays in alignment. Unless you purchase a special light-therapy lamp, you need natural light for a circadian benefit. The lights within our homes, even bright ones, are nowhere near bright enough to guide your circadian rhythm. Ideally, you want at least thirty minutes of sunlight exposure. The earlier in the morning you can get it, the better! If you are not up early enough to get morning exposure (shift workers), early afternoon light will also help. Write down how you will get your light exposure.

In the morning, I will get some sunlight by: _____

_____

In the early afternoon, I will go outside to: _____

_____

Nighttime Anxiety and Bedtime Avoidance

You may be thinking, *I feel sleepy. But when I get into bed, I am wide awake!* This is when you feel "tired but wired." Nighttime anxiety is a major culprit in the cycle of nightmares. You likely struggle with bedtime due to anxiety that works against your biology. If you are a trauma survivor, hyperarousal may happen as your body's fight-or-flight system overrides the sleep drive.

The behaviors you start trying to help this anxiety can backfire! You have probably made changes to your bedtime routine and sleep habits to try to reduce nightmares. Some are recommended (like getting out of bed if you cannot sleep) because they provide long-term benefits. Other changes may work in the short term (like keeping lights on to feel safer or sleeping in the next day to make up for lost sleep), but they have detrimental effects on sleep. Let's continue looking at how the sleep-wake cycle can get your sleep back on track and reduce nightmares.

Nightmare Avoidance Behaviors That Disrupt Sleep

With your nightmares, and especially if you have experienced trauma and have trauma-related nightmares, you probably engage in some of these avoidance behaviors. Here are common ways people relate to nightmare anxiety. Check all the ones you recognize.

THE NIGHTMARE & SLEEP DISORDER TOOLKIT

- ☐ Checking doors, windows, or security cameras multiple times before bed and/or when you wake up
- ☐ Distracting with sound (a fan, music, television)
- ☐ Sleeping with a light on
- ☐ Drinking water or other liquids to ensure you wake up
- ☐ Setting alarms to avoid nightmares
- ☐ Sleeping with a weapon
- ☐ Sleeping fully clothed
- ☐ Not sleeping in a bed
- ☐ Drinking alcohol or using other substances to fall asleep
- ☐ Using coffee or caffeine to stay awake in the evening
- ☐ Sleeping during the day instead of at night

If any of these sounds familiar, you may want to focus on changing some over the next week or two. You do not have to change everything all at once, just choose one or two. Most people find it helpful to try changing these behaviors in stages instead of all at once. Remember John the combat veteran who struggled with trauma-related nightmares for forty years? He frequently slept with the lights on to feel safer. However, this also made getting quality sleep more difficult. Here is John's plan to reduce the lighting in his room over several weeks. He also took notes about how he felt and his sleep quality over time.

John's Plan to Change His Safety Behavior

Week 1	Turn off the overhead light. Leave on two bedside lamps, the bathroom light, and the hallway light. Keep all doors open.
Week 2	Turn off the bedside lamp next to me. Leave on the far bedside lamp, bathroom light (with the door open), and the hallway light (with the door open).

Week 3	Turn off both bedside lamps. Leave on bathroom light (with the door open) and hallway lights (with the door open).
Week 4	Turn off both bedside lamps. Leave on bathroom and hallway lights but close the doors halfway.
Week 5	Turn off all lights, except for small nightlights in the hallway and bathroom only.
Week 6 and after	Ongoing maintenance.

By week 5, John was feeling really confident about turning off more lights. But he still wanted small nightlights for when he gets up to visit the bathroom. He recognized that turning on the full bathroom light at night might hurt his sleep, but he did not want to fall! With small steps, John gradually saw that he could manage nights with less light.

Consider the items on the checklist that you are willing to change. Some items might be easier than others and some might need fewer steps. For example, you might set a goal of stopping caffeine after 2 p.m. Or you might decide to try sleeping less during the day. Write your goals and any helpful notes here.

_____

_____

_____

_____

_____

_____

_____

Addressing Avoidance and Safety Behaviors

Avoidance and safety behaviors can reduce some anxiety in the short run, but in the long run they continue to reinforce the idea that you need to do the behavior to reduce danger. When you avoid things, it actually leads to an increase in anxiety as the feared item becomes even more frightening. Greater anxiety is associated with increases in nightmares. When you expect to have a nightmare, you may experience *anticipatory anxiety;* that is, the closer it gets to bedtime, the more anxious you become, and also the more likely it is that you will have nightmares. Does this sound familiar? If so, let's examine how that anxiety occurs for you.

Think about three ways you might experience nightmare-related anxiety.

- *Physiological*—how your body feels.
- *Behavioral*—what you do to try to escape the anxious feeling.
- *Cognitive*—what we tell ourselves about sleep and nightmares.

Circle all the ways you experience nightmare-related anxiety.

Physiological (in your body):

Racing heart	Anxiety	Fidgeting
Sweating	Fear	Pacing
Shortness of breath	Restlessness	Urge to move

Behavioral (in your actions):

Tossing and turning	Sleeping in clothes	Reading
Watching television	Sleeping with a weapon	Scrolling on your phone
Drinking alcohol	Sleeping with lights on	Calling a loved one
Eating	Needing a loved one to be present	Smoking

Cognitive (in your thoughts):

If I stay up later, I won't have a nightmare.	If I don't go to sleep, I won't make it through the day tomorrow.	Having nightmares means something is wrong with me.
I'm in danger in my nightmares.	Not sleeping (well) is impacting my health.	I will never recover.
I can catch up on sleep tomorrow (during the daytime).	I need to protect myself.	I need to protect my family.

Because nighttime anxiety is a major culprit in the cycle of nightmares, you will want to reduce the likelihood that it will occur. Many people who have nightmares make changes to their bedtime routines and sleep habits to reduce their experience of nightmares. Some of these changes are recommended because they provide long-term benefits. But others do not help because although they may work in the short term, they can have other detrimental effects on sleep.

Circle the number next to each item below if you have engaged in the behavior while trying to prevent having a nightmare.

1. Go to bed and wake up at the same time every day (including weekends).
2. Use a television or scroll on my phone in the bedroom.
3. Keep my bedroom cool, dark, and quiet.
4. Take naps during the day, because it is easier (or safer) to sleep in the day.
5. Exercise in the morning or early afternoon.
6. Use alcohol or tobacco before bed.
7. Use white noise machines or earplugs to reduce noise at night.
8. Use coffee and caffeine to help me stay awake in the evening.
9. Engage in quiet, calming activities one to two hours before bed.

10. Keep lights on in the bedroom all night.

11. Practice relaxation techniques right before bed or while I'm in bed.

12. Try not to have nightmares.

All the odd numbers are "Dos"—things that we recommend to help with sleep. Number one is the most important. Keep in mind that this list of things to do is only one element in this larger program to help nightmares. In fact, you may have already tried to implement these skills and are thinking, *I already did all those things!*

Just like taking multivitamins or getting regular exercise improves physical health, the odd-numbered items will improve sleep health. However, your primary care doctor would not recommend vitamins or exercise alone to treat an infection. You also need more elements from this program to improve your resistance to nightmares and overall sleep quality.

Tips for How You Can Change Sleep Habits

View this step as an experiment. The following strategies will be built into a larger treatment program. You can personalize them and try the things that you are willing or able to do. You may wonder how exercise makes a difference in sleep, or perhaps you can't do it in the morning, and the evening is the only time when you can exercise. You could experiment by moving exercise times earlier for a few weeks and tracking if it has any impact on your sleep. Or you may decide it isn't possible to change your schedule, and exercise remains important for you, so you'd rather complete it late in the day than not at all. Therefore, changing your exercise would not go on your plan.

Read these dos and don'ts. See if there is anything you might like to change about your sleep habits.

Do: Go to bed and wake up at the same time every day (including weekends).

Have you ever been on a good sleep schedule, when you wake up just a few minutes before your alarm goes off? Your body's natural clock is amazing. It's a key asset in regulating your sleep. However, it can only be helpful if it knows what to expect. Having a consistent bed and wake time is like setting your body's alarm clock so it knows when you should be tired, when you should awaken, and when it needs to build in the sleep in the middle!

Do: Keep my bedroom cool, dark, and quiet.

In REM sleep (the stage of sleep when we dream), your body is not able to *thermoregulate*, which means it can't control its temperature. Because of this, your body temperature naturally declines during REM sleep. A room that once felt warm and cozy suddenly feels hot and sweaty! Awakenings result. You can support your body's natural temperature by making sure the bedroom is cool, but still comfortable. Then when you enter REM sleep, what once felt comfortable and cool will feel warm and cozy. Body temperature can be impacted by changes across the lifespan, including medical conditions, perimenopause, or medications. Talk to your doctor if you're noticing night sweats or hot flashes. Some commercially available products may be helpful, like room fans or bedding and pajamas with moisture-wicking fabric.

We also need darkness for sleep. This can be difficult for nightmare sufferers. Leaving lights on may make you feel safer, but light signals your brain to be awake. Wherever possible, minimize light exposure during the night. This may take some time to get used to, so you may need to slowly dim the amount of light before working up to making your room completely dark. You may decide you always need a nightlight or a light on in an adjacent room (especially if you are worried about falls on the way to the bathroom or need to provide care to others at night), which is okay.

Do: Exercise in the morning or early afternoon.

Exercise is wonderful for sleep. Not only is it good for your body, but it helps you burn off energy and increase your homeostatic sleep drive so that at bedtime you are on empty and ready for a full night of sleep! However, when you exercise at night it's not helpful and possibly even harmful for your sleep. Exercising is an active process, so it signals your body that it's time to be awake and not be asleep. Doing it too close to bedtime makes calming down and going to sleep much harder. Because of this, we recommend exercising ideally in the morning or early afternoon. At the very least, do it several hours before bed. This will give your body time to relax and come back down to normal before bedtime.

Do: Use white noise machines or earplugs to reduce noise at night.

You may have heard of "things that go bump in the night." When you hear a sound but there is no apparent cause, you can lie in bed wondering what on earth it was. You can become anxious and even get up to check or rummage through the house looking for the cause. These sounds are likely unavoidable. You may live in a city, share your home with family members, or have pets who are active at night. For this reason, running a white noise machine, wearing earplugs, or turning on a fan can help produce a more peaceful environment. You are less likely to be disturbed by the sounds that naturally occur during the night.

Do: Engage in quiet, calming activities one to two hours before bed.

Having a wind-down routine, a series of steps you complete every night before bed, can signal to your body that it is time to sleep. You may already do this without recognizing it's setting the stage for bedtime. A nighttime hygiene routine, such as brushing teeth, washing your face, and visiting the restroom, often precede bedtime. These are examples of stimulus control, as pre-bedtime activities can prime your body and brain to be ready for sleep. These activities will not cause you to go to sleep. Sleep is a biological process like hunger, so we cannot create sleepiness. But you can do things to encourage it, like a wind-down routine.

Sarah realized she was spending the hour before bed doing activating things, like running on her treadmill, watching an action series, and sometimes having heated discussions with her spouse. All this discouraged sleep. So she changed her routine. Now, an hour before bed, Sarah dims the lights in the house. Then she performs the same routine each night: changing into nightclothes, washing her face, brushing her teeth, praying. This helps her body relax and recognize bedtime.

What do you currently do in the hour before bed?

_____

_____

_____

How do these activities discourage your body from sleeping or promote sleep?

_____

_____

_____

_____

Let's not forget the even-numbered items! We do not recommend them. If you are using some of these elements, consider reducing the number of items. You may also choose to not change any of these elements right now, and that is okay. We want you to make changes you are willing to make across this program.

Don't: Use a television or scroll on my phone in the bedroom.

This is one of the most unpopular recommendations on the list, but it's among the most important. First, recall stimulus control and limiting the bed (and ideally the entire bedroom) to sleep and sexual activity. Watching television or scrolling on your phone will only pair your bedroom with being awake. Further, both television and your phone emit stimulating blue light. Your television gives off much less, so we would recommend not streaming on a phone or tablet. Even better, do it in a separate room and not in your bedroom!

Don't: Take naps during the day, because it's easier (or safer) to sleep in the day.

Another unpopular recommendation is not to nap during the day. It makes sense to make up for lost sleep if you are sleep deprived and also to sleep during the time you feel safest. However, consider your homeostatic sleep drive: The more you nap during the day, the more you reduce your drive to sleep at night. This often makes it more difficult to fall and stay asleep. Further, napping during the day happens in a brighter environment, which leads to a less restful sleep. As difficult as it is, try to avoid napping when possible. If you do nap, limit it to a thirty-minute power nap before three o'clock in the afternoon. This is enough sleep to give you some energy in the afternoon. But you won't wake up wanting to sleep more, feeling worse than you did when you went to sleep!

Don't: Use alcohol or tobacco before bed.

Some people report using alcohol to relax. They say it shortens the amount of time it takes to fall asleep. However, we know that alcohol changes *sleep architecture*—the stages of sleep throughout the night. Alcohol may help you fall asleep initially, but it reduces the amount of slow-wave sleep. This results in less refreshing sleep and more sleep fragmentation, which makes it more likely you'll wake up. Additionally, drinking any liquid before bed can increase the need to use the restroom, which further disrupts sleep. With increased sleep fragmentation, alcohol can make nightmares more likely in the second half of the night. These are all reasons to limit the alcohol you consume close to bedtime.

Nicotine, found in tobacco, is a stimulant. Stimulants make it harder to sleep, so avoiding tobacco and nicotine products before bed is a good recommendation for most people. But withdrawal symptoms from tobacco may also worsen sleep. Experiment on your own, if you use these products. For example, try moving your last use to an hour before bed for a week. Track this on your sleep diary. After the week, are there any changes? Notice when you are using nicotine and how it may impact your sleep. If you are interested in quitting, talk to your healthcare provider about options.

Don't: Use coffee or caffeine to help you stay awake in the evening.

Do you use coffee or caffeine to keep yourself up at night? Many people with nightmares avoid sleep in order to avoid nightmares. *Avoiding sleep actually makes nightmares more likely.* We do not recommend it. We encourage you to experiment with your caffeine use. Caffeine has a four- to six-hour half-life. That means it can take four to six hours for the caffeine in your system to reduce by half. Experiment with cutting off your caffeine by noon or 2 p.m. (or ten hours before bedtime). For a week, reduce or move your last cup of coffee (or tea, or other caffeinated beverage of choice) to earlier in the day. Track it in your sleep diary. If your sleep changes, consider making a long-term change. If you do not notice any difference, you could return to using it.

Don't: Keep lights on in the bedroom all night.

Do you feel safer with a lot of lights on when you are trying to sleep? Or maybe it feels safer if you wake up to immediately see your bedroom. This is a *safety behavior*, which you may do to feel more secure. But it may make things worse. It's is likely reducing your sleep quality. For the same reason we encourage light exposure in the daytime, we discourage light exposure in the evening. Try experimenting with reducing the amount of light in your bedroom over time to see if it helps your sleep quality. Earlier in the chapter, we included John's plan for doing this, which you can adapt to your own needs.

From the list of dos and don'ts, try to pick something you'd be willing to try in the next week.

I am willing to try adding: _____

I am willing to reduce: _____

What are some of the reasons why making this change is important to you?

_____

_____

_____

_____

_____

All the recommendations in this chapter can be personalized according to your plan and needs. Choose the changes that will be support you. We hope this review of evidence-based strategies offered you clear rationales for how they promote healthy sleep, so you're more likely to engage in them consistently. In the next chapter, we'll share one of the most effective tools for sleeping well.

CHAPTER 6

Relaxation

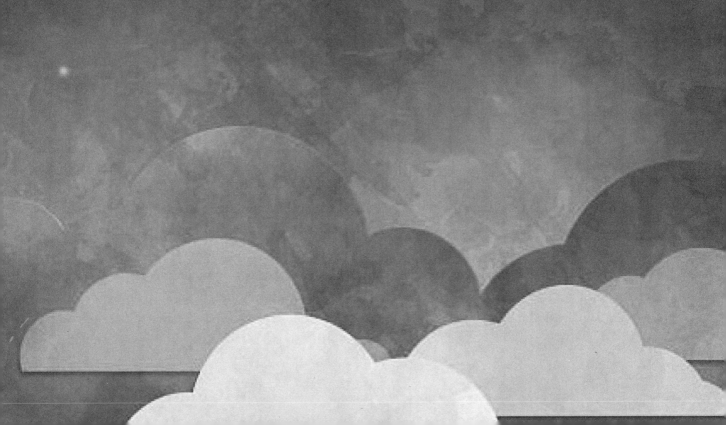

THE NIGHTMARE & SLEEP DISORDER TOOLKIT

With your sleep problems, you may have difficulty relaxing. Especially when sleeping in a bed has become associated with some difficult experiences like nightmares. It's helpful to learn some relaxation practices to address your level of *physiological arousal*—how alert and awake your body is during the day and at night. If you are anxious at bedtime, you are more likely to have worse sleep quality and more nightmares. Having nightmares on one night predicts the likelihood you will have another nightmare the next night. Remember this cycle:

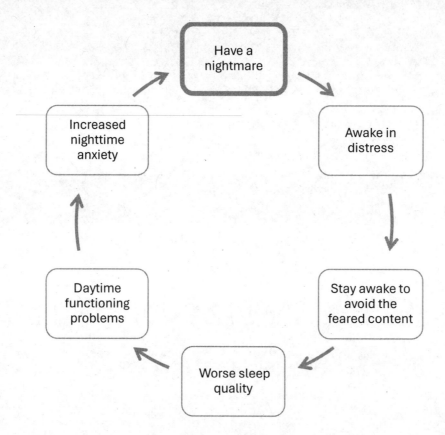

This book provides different tools to help break this cycle at multiple points! Relaxation is incompatible with anxiety—if you get your body into a relaxed state, your mind will follow. Reducing the amount of anxiety you feel at bedtime is one step closer to breaking the nightmare cycle. Also, relaxation will help most with daytime functioning problems and the nighttime anxiety. When we increase relaxation, we reduce anxiety and distress. In doing so, we can help break the loop of anxiety. In this chapter, we'll explore two relaxation strategies that you might use to address this: deep breathing and progressive muscle relaxation (PMR). We'll share how your mood at bedtime may tend to match the mood in your dreams, and help you get started, track progress, and gauge the effects of relaxation on your nightmares.

Deep Breathing

When we take in breaths rapidly and very shallowly, we can create more anxiety. If you've ever hyperventilated, you know this feeling! The opposite—exhaling slowly and completely between breaths—brings relaxation to our parasympathetic nervous system. Here's a quick exercise you can try now to check in with your breathing.

Lay this book down on a table or armrest. Put one hand on your chest and one hand right below your breastbone, at the top of your stomach. At first, don't try to do anything differently. Just breathe as you normally would and notice the movement, or lack of movement, in your hands. Your chest is rising and falling. If your stomach hand is moving it all, it's much less than your chest. This exercise tends to show that people breathe shallower (in their chest) throughout the day.

Now notice how your body is feeling and its level of stress or tension. Using the Subjective Units of Distress Scale (SUDS), rate your stress. On a 0 to 10 scale, 0 is calm and relaxed, and 10 is the most distress you can feel. Write your SUDS, as follows.

Rate how you are feeling right now. _____

Rate how you felt waking up from your most recent nightmare. _____

Hopefully these numbers are different! Your SUDS levels vary throughout the day. However, most people find that their SUDS levels increase when faced with a stressor. If you are a trauma survivor, it might be hard to think of a recent time when your SUDS level was at a 0 on the scale. People with nightmares, from any source, usually have greater distress during the day. Working to reduce your baseline SUDS level through relaxation can help reduce the likelihood of nightmares. It can also reduce the daytime symptoms like irritability and difficulty concentrating.

To bring on relaxation, work on taking some deeper breaths. The opposite, breathing quickly and shallowly (hyperventilating), signals danger and activation. Signal your body to relax by increasing the flow of oxygen and breathing slowly. Next you'll learn a deep-breathing exercise that can bring on a relaxation response. A guided audio recording is available at https://www.newharbinger.com/55817.

Take note of your SUDS level before starting this exercise. _____

Exercise for Deep Breathing

As before, place your hands on your chest and belly. Begin to take slower and deeper breaths, expanding down into the belly. Watching the rise of your chest, on the next inhale, try to breathe in so deeply that your belly expands. Take a couple of breaths this way. It may feel uncomfortable or unfamiliar at first, so we're going to work on breathing in a relaxing way next.

Take a breath in and *inhale* through your nose for a count of 2, then *exhale* for a count of 4, and then *pause* for a count of 2. Just pause—don't hold your breath. Then start the next inhale and follow the same counts.

Try to repeat this for a cycle of ten breaths: *Breathe in for 2, out for 4, and pause for 2, before inhaling again.*

After ten breaths, return to breathing normally and notice how your body feels.

Compared to the start of the exercise, does it feel the same or different? Write what you notice. Perhaps your shoulders are lower, your back is not as tense, you have less anxiety.

_____

_____

_____

_____

Rate that SUDS level again on a 0 to 10 scale, where 0 is relaxed, and 10 is the most distressed you could be.

SUDS = _____

Is the level lower than your rating at the start of this section? If so, great!

You may notice a small decrease. You might still feel distressed but feel less tension in your body. Or there won't be any change the first time you try the exercise. If you were so focused on trying to learn the new skill, you may not be bringing on relaxation. If there was no change, you can still benefit from this exercise. You just need more practice!

Practice, Practice, Practice

Practicing deep breathing over time can help bring on a relaxation response. Lots of valuable resources online offer recordings for practicing. You can also find a guided audio recording at https://www.newharbinger.com/55817. Most people find it helpful to listen to a recording when they practice. Over time, the exercise becomes more natural and you may not need the recording. We recommend you practice deep breathing twice per day, for ten to fifteen minutes, for a week. Then you'll develop some confidence in your ability to bring on the relaxation response. Think about when you'd like to practice. Some people do it first thing in the morning, at lunch, or during a scheduled break in their day.

I plan to practice:

Date and time: _____

First practice session: _____

Second practice session: _____

Deep breathing is portable and discreet, as you do not have to use the hand placements. Many people find it easy to use across situations. It is not a skill *only* to reduce anxiety related to sleep and nightmares. Feel free to use it whenever you notice your SUDS levels are a little higher, your shoulders a bit more tense, or you are having negative thoughts.

Progressive Muscle Relaxation (PMR)

PMR is a whole-body exercise designed to bring on relaxation. It tenses and releases each major muscle group to relieve tension. However, you may have pain or injuries where muscle tension would not be helpful. For example, if you have pain in your back, visualize this area but do not tense those muscles during the exercise.

You do not want to squeeze too hard, so tense your muscles between 25 to 50 percent of the maximum tension. You may like to complete this exercise lying down, but you can also do it while sitting in a comfortable position.

Start by rating your SUDS level. Remember: 0 = relaxed; 10 = the most distress you can feel.

SUDS = _____

Exercise for Progressive Muscle Relaxation

Plan to spend ten to fifteen minutes on this exercise, in a space where you can be free from distractions.

Step 1: Place one hand on your chest and one hand on your belly. Just breathe in and out as you normally would, inhaling and exhaling. Notice how your hands move as you breathe, with one hand moving slightly more than the other. As we work through this exercise, breathe more deeply and slowly. Take a deep breath again. See if you can make the lower hand on your belly move. Work on filling up your belly with air. Then exhale slowly, feeling it collapse. Take a couple more breaths: In through your nose and out through your mouth. Observe the rise and fall of your breath. Continue this throughout the progressive muscle relaxation.

In the coming steps, we are going to move through different muscle groups in your body. You'll focus on each one, tensing and releasing each muscle group. As you tense and release, try to picture that muscle group tensing and releasing. You can close your eyes to help picture the muscle groups, or if you are not comfortable with that, soften your gaze and focus on a single space. If you have areas of pain, only do the imagery part and don't physically tense and release those muscles. Then rejoin the exercise, tensing the next group where you feel comfortable.

Step 2: Breathe in. As you do, raise your eyebrows as if they could touch the top of your forehead. Picture those tense muscles in your forehead, and then release. Notice the softness in your face as that tension goes away. Breathe in and out. Move down to your eyes, squinting them tight so no light can get in. Notice the muscles around your eyes as you hold for 5-4-3-2-1. Then release, letting your eyes relax. Appreciate the softness in your face. Move down to your mouth and raise up the corners like you're smiling. Feel the cheek muscles tense as you hold for 5-4-3-2-1, and release. Take a few breaths here, in and out. Appreciate the softness in your face, noticing how those muscles feel more relaxed than they did when you started.

Step 3: Move down into your neck. As a reminder if you have pain, only picture the muscles—don't tense them. Tilt your neck up toward the ceiling. Notice the muscles in your throat tighten as you hold for 5-4-3-2-1, and release. Let your neck fall back to a neutral position. If you want, twist or roll the neck a bit to notice the looseness. Now for the opposite. Drop your chin down to your chest, feeling the muscles in the back of your neck tighten as you hold for 5-4-3-2-1, and release. Notice the sense of relaxation, from the top of your head down to your neck. Notice the softness. Take another breath and exhale. Continue breathing in and out as you move down your body.

Step 4: Lift your shoulders up to tense your muscles for 5-4-3-2-1, and release. Let your shoulders drop down. Feel your arms hanging limp at your sides. Notice the sense of softness, the sense of relaxation. Then take your arms and pull up, like you're flexing your biceps as you hold for 5-4-3-2-1, and release. Let your arms hang limp at your side, noticing the difference. Put your arms out in front of you, locking your elbows and tensing the muscles of your forearms for 5-4-3-2-1, and release. Breathe in and out. Roll your shoulders and let those arms fall gently at your side, appreciating the softness in your body and the sense of relaxation as you breathe in and out.

Step 5: Move down into your chest. Take a deep breath, hold it for 5-4-3-2-1, and release those chest muscles back down. Move into the back, pulling those shoulder blades so they come back toward your spine as you hold tight for 5-4-3-2-1, and release. Breathe in and out for a couple of breaths. Moving down into the abdomen, in the belly, take a deep breath. Let that abdomen expand and hold it for 5-4-3-2-1, and release. Take a regular breath, in and out, and then take a deep breath in and out. Now move the belly button toward the spine, tightening those abdominal muscles and picturing them squeezing for 5-4-3-2-1, and release. Take a couple deep breaths as you notice the sense of relaxation that starts at the top of your head, comes down through your body, out through your arms, and into your chest. Take a deep breath, in and out, before you move into the lower body.

Step 6: Squeeze your butt together, picturing those large muscles tightening as you hold for 5-4-3-2-1, and release. Move down into your quadriceps. Pull your knees together and tighten those upper leg muscles. Picture those muscles tightening as if holding a penny between your knees and hold for 5-4-3-2-1, and release. Let the hips fall apart a little bit, dropping those knees. Move into the legs, pointing your toes to tighten those calf muscles as you hold for 5-4-3-2-1, and release. Now go the opposite way, bringing toes back to your shinbones for 5-4-3-2-1, and release. You may want to roll your ankles here. Stretch however feels good, taking a few deep breaths. The last set is your toes. Curl them under, gently holding for 5-4-3-2-1, and release. Wiggle those toes and wiggle those feet, if you need to.

Step 6: As you breathe in and out, let waves of relaxation start at the top of your head, run down through your body, and go out through your toes. You may feel warmth or lightness or tingling. Notice how relaxation has moved through your entire body during the exercise.

Record your SUDS level on a scale of 0 to 10. SUDS = _____

You can read through the exercise as many times as you need. Start with ten- to fifteen-minute practices, which fit into your busy life. There are much longer scripts, even up to forty-five minutes, that some people enjoy. We encourage you to practice with a script or recording at first. Read this script, or a similar one, to yourself aloud as you work through each section. If it's difficult to both relax and read the script, ask a loved one to read it aloud for the first several practices. You can also find an audio recording of it at https://www.newharbinger.com/55817. In addition, there are many valuable resources available as mobile apps and online. Over time, as the exercise becomes more natural, you may not need the recording.

Practice, Practice, Practice

Practicing progressive muscle relaxation will build confidence. It can help reduce your daytime anxiety, which will help reduce a factor that contributes to nightmares. Think about when you would like to practice. Some people like to use this first thing in the morning, during a scheduled break in their day, or as part of their nighttime wind-down routine.

I plan to practice:

Date and time: _____

First practice session: _____

Second practice session: _____

The goal is to help reduce daytime distress and nighttime anxiety, as increased distress and anxiety can prime your body to be more likely to experience nightmares. PMR is less portable than deep breathing, but may bring deeper relaxation. Practice both, noticing which one works for you. You can use these skills at different times in your day, for different reasons. For example, use deep breathing before a meeting at work, then use PMR in the evening when you have more time to work on relaxation. Experiment with what works for you and your lifestyle.

Why Does Anxiety Increase Nightmares?

Some scientists propose that nightmares may be partially related to something called *mood matching*. The mood matching theory suggests that our mood at bedtime can influence our dreams and nightmares (Mallett et al. 2022). This is often heard in popular advice cautioning against watching scary movies at bedtime. There's truth to this idea. Our mood at bedtime can influence dreams and nightmares. This is a reason we focus on daytime distress and nighttime anxiety in nightmare treatment.

Think about this like a radio or music app. When you're playing music, you often select music to fit your mood. You play something catchy for an upbeat mood and something slower or angrier to match sadness or frustration. Sometimes your mood might change before you notice that the song has changed. You might be driving and find yourself gripping the steering wheel tighter or yelling at other drivers, and then notice a super-annoying song is playing. The song influenced your mood (irritability) and your behavior (gripping steering wheel). Hopefully you changed the song before you started speeding or driving aggressively!

You may experience sleep problems, including nightmares, when you are anxious or upset at bedtime. This anxiety can make nightmares more likely. Do you notice that you're feeling anxious or upset at bedtime?

Check your recent sleep diaries for nights when the bedtime anxiety ratings were higher. What else did you notice on those nights?

_____

_____

_____

_____

Nighttime anxiety may impact your sleep in the following ways:

- More difficulty falling asleep
- More nighttime awakenings
- Feeling less rested in the morning
- More nightmares
- Higher nightmare frequency or intensity

On nights when you recorded higher levels of distress in your sleep diary, were you more likely to have nightmares?

Circle one: **Yes   No**

Working on nighttime anxiety can be important for improving sleep and nightmares. Some people notice that nighttime anxiety is associated with the bed or bedroom specifically. You might say, "I fall asleep on the couch no problem, but when I get in bed, I can't fall asleep." Or, "I feel sleepy getting into bed, but then I'm wide awake in bed." Does that sound familiar?

This workbook aims to reduce sleep-related anxiety that stems from both fear of nightmares and failed past attempts to correct sleep disturbances. Training in sleep hygiene practices and relaxation can start to undo pairing your bed (or bedroom) with anxiety.

Your Ongoing Relaxation Practice

You previously decided *when* you plan on practicing, but we thought it may be good to process *why* you'll practice relaxation going forward. Like any skill, the more you practice relaxation, and the more purposeful your practice, the better the results will be. Think back on the practice you have done, and the success you have had, to consider how the practice will help move you toward your goals.

Relaxation practice is going to help me reach my goals by: _____

_____

_____

_____

_____

Are there any ways you can make this practice more likely? You could set a reminder in your phone, put a sticky note in a frequently visited location, or ask a loved one for help remembering to practice this skill daily. Write these down.

_____

_____

_____

_____

_____

You'll want to add this practice to your sleep and nightmare log. You can start to see the effects of your practice by noticing any changes in your sleep or nightmares when you practice. So add the following questions to your sleep and nightmare logs.

Date				
Did you practice relaxation techniques during the day? (Y/N)				
Did you practice relaxation techniques right before bed, or in bed? (Y/N)				
Did you engage in quiet, calming activities in the hours before bed? (Y/N)				

You can also download an updated sleep and nightmare diary for repeated use at https://www.newharbinger.com/55817.

Once you have practiced a few times, consider your relaxation practice. Because treatments for sleep problems are most effective when used in the hours surrounding sleep, practice is important. We know making changes to your sleep can be difficult.

How many days and nights were you able to practice a relaxation strategy? Choose one.

☐ 0: I didn't start (I didn't want to).

☐ 1 to 2: I tried it.

☐ 3 to 4: I practiced a few times this week.

☐ 5 to 7: I practiced regularly.

What did you like about relaxation? What did you not like?

___

___

___

Now consider whether relaxation practice made any changes in your daytime functioning or bedtime anxiety ratings. Reflect on the days you practiced. Did you see changes in how you felt during the day? Were there changes in your bedtime anxiety?

_____

_____

_____

_____

_____

The part of the relaxation practice that was the easiest for me was _____

because _____.

The part of the relaxation assignment that was most difficult was _____

because _____.

Things that may help me in overcome the difficulty I had with relaxation practice are: (Circle all that apply or write your own.)

Asking a loved one for help	Setting a reminder on my phone	Looking at my goals and how this will help	Using an audio recording	Scheduling practice
Writing a sticky note reminder	Taking time on my lunch break	Finding a different script	Writing (rewriting) my exercise	Trying a different relaxation skill
Asking a loved one to practice with me	Keeping my eyes open during practice	Closing my eyes during practice	Using headphones	

Other: _____ _____

_____ _____

In these initial chapters, you began working on three of the four elements in the nightmare cycle to improve sleep quality through:

1. Sleep hygiene (keeping a consistent bedtime, for example)

2. Stimulus control (like using the bed only for sleep and sex)

3. Managing daytime distress and nighttime anxiety (practicing relaxation through deep breathing or progressive muscle relaxation)

Working steadily to make changes in each domain begins to break up the nightmare cycle. These changes are usually gradual. Looking at your sleep and nightmare logs, you will likely notice changes—maybe small decreases in your bedtime anxiety ratings. Or you are getting up at the same time every day. You may receive feedback from a bed partner or other loved one about your sleep or daytime distress, as you're less irritable or more energetic. If you're already seeing changes, great! If not, remember these changes are usually gradual. It's likely you're seeing minimal changes and wondering, *But what about my nightmares?* Nightmares are a learned behavior, and it takes time to unlearn them! In the next chapter we'll start addressing them directly.

CHAPTER 7

Visualization

You are ready to learn a powerful skill to directly attack your nightmares: visualization! Up to this point, the skills have aimed to reduce nightmares by improving your sleep and laying the foundation. Now you can directly address your nightmare problem. Visualization is a core skill in IRT because, in many ways, it's the one responsible for changing a nightmare into a dream that you select. In this chapter, you'll learn visualization. Then in chapter 8, you'll tailor your visualization to target the nightmares!

Visualization is a vital tool for fixing your nightmare circle. It directly affects the nightmare by changing it to a dream you would like to have. This also improves sleep quality because there is less reason to awaken in the absence of a nightmare, which improves your daytime functioning, reduces anxiety, and lowers your chances of having nightmares in the future.

How Visualization Works

Nightmares are visual pictures. They come from a part of your brain called the *visual cortex*. This visual cortex is more active during sleep than other areas of your brain. For example, your *prefrontal cortex* handles *executive control*—using logic to make decisions. When asleep, you don't have much control over what the visual and emotional centers of your brain do. However, while you're awake, you can train this visual system! Training it, and practicing while awake, strengthens this neural pathway. Then it's more likely that your brain will choose to play a non-nightmare visualization at night. For most people, this strategy takes a good bit of practice.

Ever heard of elite athletes using visualization as a tool to help improve performance? They develop a very vivid picture of successfully executing their sport in their mind's eye. Before a competition, they walk through the visualization using sights, sounds, smells, and all senses. You may have seen athletes doing this. For example, a hurdler might walk onto the track, feel the ground change, pay attention to the lighting and the smell of the arena. Then they picture themselves setting up in their stance, listening for the cue to start, and their arms and legs moving during the event.

Picturing yourself moving through skills or tasks before performing them can aid in performance (Porter 2003). There is evidence this makes changes in the brain, as it activates the *mirror neurons*. These are brain cells that fire when we watch someone else performing a task, so we can learn by watching others. These *ventral premotor cortex cells* fire when we perform an action—and when we watch someone act. This is how watching others may help prime your brain for when you later try the same task. Visualization may work the same way, as picturing yourself performing a task may improve future performance on those tasks.

When trying to train your brain to have a new dream, practicing this dream content while you're awake helps prime the brain to dream it overnight.

Exercise for Visualization

Let's start with a simple exercise. Visualize eating a piece of chocolate cake. You may already have a favorite slice of cake in mind. It may have icing, sprinkles, or chocolate flavoring. See the layers of alternating cake and frosting. Close your eyes and try to picture the slice of cake in front of you. Then open your eyes and read on.

Did you see it? If so, try to add even more detail to your visualization. If you struggled a bit, that's okay. This is a new skill, or maybe chocolate cake isn't for you. You could try again with a different favorite food!

Now try taking a bite! Use your imagination to cut into that same cake with a fork. Imagine yourself taking a bite. Notice what sensations you experience. Close your eyes to picture it.

Are you hungry now? Depending on the vividness of the image, you may even notice salivation. Or you may think about where you can get a slice of cake. The more sensory details you can include in the imagery, the more your visual cortex will be activated.

This can apply to nightmares. You may be thinking, *I don't want my nightmares to be more vivid!* We don't either! We are talking about visualization for two reasons.

Relaxation: If you tried the progressive muscle relaxation in the last chapter, recall how you visualized muscle groups. That was called *guided imagery,* another form of relaxation that we'll soon explore.

Nightmare Rescription: One of the strongest interventions for nightmares is to rescript them, from a scary and distressing event to something neutral or pleasant. This supplies the visual system of the brain with different imagery, so when it begins to call up a dream, it has different options or pathways.

How Visualization Treats Nightmares

Think about your dreams as if you're going on a hike through the woods. You're on a path that is clear, well-maintained, and gets visited frequently. This is your brain's current nightmare trail. Just as nightmares are a learned behavior, your brain has been practicing hiking this trail for a while. You're tired of hiking to this lookout, as the trail and view are scary. But because it's such a well-worn pathway, your brain goes down that pathway by default. In fact, your brain may not even see any options. As you read this paragraph, you may have been picturing what the nightmare trail looks like. That's visualization!

Using imagery, we're going to work on creating a new trail through the woods. It'll take time for the new trail to be as clear and well-maintained as the old one. You can choose what the path looks like, the scenic viewpoint, and the destination. Join us on a pleasant walk in the woods now. As you picture this pleasant walk in the woods, engage your senses. Here are some examples of questions you might ask for each of the five senses.

1. **Sight:** What colors do you see? What types of trees, grasses, or flowers do you notice? Are there rocks?

2. **Sound:** Can you hear the wind? What about birds? Is there a river nearby or in the distance?

3. **Touch:** Can you feel a breeze? Maybe you reach out to touch a flower or some tree bark.

4. **Smell:** Are you in a pine forest? Are there fragrant flowers? Can you smell the dirt?

5. **Taste:** (This one might be harder.) Do you stop to enjoy wild blackberries or taste the coffee you packed in a thermos?

Here is an example script of walking in the woods. Engage your senses as you read through this sample visualization.

> I tighten the straps on my backpack and make sure my shoes are tied as I check the trail map one more time. I see an opening in the woods with a clearly marked path. I'm feeling excited about this hike because I know there are some great views ahead, I can smell the pine trees, and it's a warm day. I feel the sun and a slight cool breeze

as I'm walking the path. I hear birds and I see a squirrel jump onto a tree limb. My legs feel strong. As I walk, I see some interesting ferns and lodgepole pines.

This trail is great! They have signs at regular intervals to ensure I'm on the right path. After walking a few minutes, I can see that there is a clearing ahead. I start to hear a stream babbling along. As I approach the clearing, I see the stream running past the trail. It's not very deep, so I can see that the bottom is rocky. On the opposite bank, I see flowers.

I take a sip of water, which feels refreshing. If I come here again, I'd like to bring my camera. I still have more trail ahead, so I start walking again. The path is clear, smooth, and well-maintained. Every now and then, I step over a root from the surrounding trees. Through the clearing, I see the path zigzagging ahead. There is another sign where maybe this trail meets another one. I continue walking, appreciating the birds chirping, the rustling of leaves, the occasional squirrel jumping branch to branch.

When I approach the sign, I know I'm going to stay on my current trail. The arrows clearly point me forward: I feel reassured and excited because I know a beautiful view is ahead. There's a slight slope as I gain elevation, but it's still an easy hike. My heart rate increases slightly with the change in elevation and the excitement. I pause one more time for a water break and check my watch. I've been hiking for about thirty minutes now and I'm very close!

I go around a big tree and see the lake overlook. It's lovely. There's a bench and plenty of space. I see one other hiker heading back down the trail and they give me a friendly wave. I settle on the bench. I plan to stay here a few moments, appreciating this view of the lake, before hiking back.

Were you able to picture the woods as you read through this script? How did it feel? Write some reflections down or make some notes for writing your own script later.

_____

_____

_____

_____

Forging a New Path

In choosing nightmare treatment, you're forging a new path through the woods. The pathway you create can take you to a different destination—a beautiful lake lookout or even the top of a waterfall. However, this path is not yet built. The woods are dense. So you're going to build a new dream that is pleasant or neutral, with lots of detail. To do this, you must tackle the obstacles and build this trail through practice. You can clear brush, haul rocks, and put up signposts. You'll do this through visualization!

To create the new path for your brain to take at night, you must engage the senses and practice this trail to help your visual system. The more you practice, the more you manicure that path, the easier it will be. With practice, as your brain approaches visual content, it can choose the visualization path instead of the nightmare path. Over time, that nightmare path will look overgrown. It won't be as easy to hike. Before you use visualization to treat your nightmares, you can learn visualization skills more generally.

Start with pleasant imagery unrelated to your nightmares. As elite athletes show, visualization helps improve performance. It can also be a relaxation strategy on its own, to reduce nighttime anxiety and daytime distress that often come with nightmares. Remember: relaxation is incompatible with anxiety. So visualization is both a relaxation strategy and a powerful tool to change nightmare content. Let's practice a full visualization exercise. Then you can choose from these different exercises for your practice sessions.

Exercise to Practice Visualization Skills

As you prepare, set the stage. Find a comfortable and quiet place. Some people like to remain sitting, and others prefer to lie down. We recommend that you close your eyes, but if this is uncomfortable, find a single spot on the ceiling, floor, or wall and soften your gaze. The first time you practice, you'll likely want to read the script below slowly or have someone read it to you. There is a guided audio recording available at https://www.newharbinger.com/55817. There are also other options online and through mobile apps that you may want to explore later.

Before we begin, rate your SUDS level: _____

Let's visit the ocean. Take several deep breaths. As you do, notice how the air coming in is cooler than the air going out. Focus on this breathing coming in and out, in and out, in and out. Scan your body to notice any areas of tension or pain, without judgment. Let yourself feel more relaxed and more comfortable, sinking into the chair or bed as you breathe in and out.

In your mind, picture being at the top of the staircase. You are going to take one step at a time, pausing to notice how the wooden steps feel under your feet. Looking ahead, you can see that at the end of the stairs, there is a beautiful sandy beach. See waves crashing on the shore, and with each step down the staircase, feel more and more tension melting away.

As you get closer, notice that the sand is not flat. It has little hills and valleys. See the shoreline stretching down the beach, seemingly going on forever in each direction. As you approach the last step, you pause to look out at the ocean. Notice how bright blue—almost turquoise—the water is and see the white caps running up against the sand.

When you take a step down into that sand, feel your feet sinking into the warmth of the sand. You get a little bit between your toes and this sensation is soothing, as you feel more and more relaxation throughout your body. You hear the roaring sound of the ocean. The waves crashing over each other provide a deep calm for your body and mind.

Start walking toward the edge of the water, noticing the warm sun on your face. There's a salty smell in the air, and you hear gulls crying in the distance. Take a deep breath, breathing in the scent of the salt air, and feel more and more relaxed. As you approach the edge of the water, you notice cool water rushing over your toes. It feels refreshing and relaxing. Stand here for a moment, watching the waves, feeling the breeze and the sun, tasting the salt air, hearing waves crash in the distance.

Stay here as long as you would like, breathing in and out. If you like, you can turn back toward the beach and find a comfortable chair. Sit down and relax, breathing in and out, feeling more and more relaxed as you settle in for a few more minutes. Stay here and let yourself enjoy looking around at this beautiful scenery. Enjoy the sights and sounds of the beach. When you feel ready, gently bring yourself back to the room, staying comfortable, staying still, staying relaxed.

Now rate your SUDS again: _____

Did you notice changes in your SUDS, bodily tension, or sense of well-being while completing this exercise? Was it awkward? Or effortless? Write about your experience.

_____
_____
_____
_____
_____
_____
_____

You may have noticed the relaxation response in this practice. If so, great! If not, you are in good company. That does not mean visualization will not work for you, it just means you need more practice! Visualization is a skill that takes time to develop.

You can use this script to practice this week. Or you can make your own. Some people don't find the beach relaxing (too much sand). If you prefer, you can drive on a country road, walk through a busy city, or enjoy a lovely meal. The content is up to you. Just keep it pleasant and detailed! Feel that sun or cool breeze. See the people, lights, or trees. Smell those pine needles, dirt roads, meat on the grill. Taste that sweet tea! Hear that music, car horns, or sizzle. Really work to engage all your senses.

Helpful Tips: Practice when you have time and space to fully engage with the visualization. Record yourself, a loved one, or find an online recording. Listening to the script can be easier than trying to read and picture it at the same time. Some people also find that listening to a recording helps them remain focused. The source is less important than the practice! You can find recordings of this exercise and a few more at https://www.newharbinger.com/55817.

If you want to make your own script, write it down here. Make sure you write down every sight, smell, sound, taste, and touch.

_____
_____
_____
_____
_____
_____
_____
_____
_____

Practicing Visualization

Let's implement that visualization! We recommend doing visualization practice twice daily. Continue to practice either deep breathing or progressive muscle relaxation. Some people like to pair these skills, while others find it helpful to complete them at different times. We recommend practicing twice daily, for ten to fifteen minutes per session.

I plan to practice: _____

_____
_____

I will do this at _____ *a.m. / p.m. (circle one)* and *at* _____ *a.m. / p.m.* (circle one).

This will help me reach my goals by: _____

_____

_____

Are there any ways you can make this practice more likely? You can set a reminder in your phone, put a sticky note in a frequently visited location, or ask a loved one for help remembering to practice this skill.

To support my visualization practice, I will: _____

_____

_____

_____

Add this practice to your sleep and nightmare logs. When you practice, you'll see the effects by noticing any change in your sleep or nightmares. You can download an updated sleep and nightmare diary at https://www.newharbinger.com/55817.

If you have been working through this book slowly, you may have already seen notable changes in your sleep. If you are moving through it a bit faster, it may be too soon. Either way, if your sleep quality has not improved, reflect back on the factors that impact sleep quality. See whether you can tweak your sleep a bit more in order to get even better results.

At this point in the workbook, you're likely experiencing improvement in some of your daytime distress and nighttime anxiety. In the coming chapters, you'll continue to learn skills that help as you start to work on the nightmares. Let's add interventions for other areas of the nightmare cycle. Here is the nightmare cycle again:

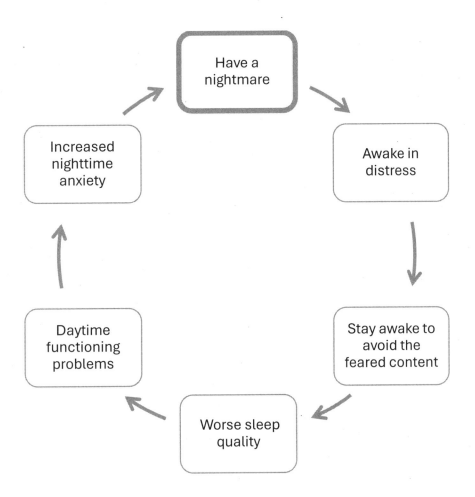

Rescription, the topic of the next chapter, works on the nightmare directly. It can also help with nighttime awakenings as you begin to feel greater control over your nightmares. If you identified rescription as part of your treatment plan, enjoy learning it next.

CHAPTER 8

Exposure and Rescription

In this chapter, we'll start to build on your visualization skills and work on your new dream. We've discussed consistent bed and wake times, and you have been practicing relaxation to reduce nighttime anxiety and daytime distress. With strategies to improve sleep quality, and by doing visualization, you may start to have dreams that are like the visualization. Or your dreams might be a mix of that content and other content. Maybe you are having fewer or less severe nightmares! As you look at your sleep diaries, notice some trends or patterns. Are you having fewer wake-ups? Is your sleep quality improved? These are all things that we want to look at. Just like building our skills practice, the results sometimes take a little time, but the stronger we get at our practice, typically the better the results are.

Types of Nightmares

Let's discuss what nightmares may look like or represent. There are usually three types of nightmares.

> **Idiopathic nightmares** do not appear to have any connection to real life or traumatic events but have upsetting content, nonetheless, with vivid sights, sounds, and emotions.
>
> **Similar or symbolic dreams** may have some of the elements of a lived experience, but then other parts do not match. An example would be a combat veteran replaying a battle, but then family members who were not present at the event show up on the battlefield. Another example is a car accident survivor dreaming of a plane crash. Alternatively, it could have similar emotions or themes to a lived experience like being threatened, feeling out of control, or being otherwise unsafe. These can be quite confusing and distressing.
>
> **Replicative nightmares** are a close replay of the event with the same sights, sounds, and emotions. Some feel stuck replaying the same distressing event, night after night. Tired of dealing with it while you sleep, you may avoid the content during the day. But this only makes the nightmare more likely to occur.
>
> Remember John, our combat veteran? His nightmare replayed a specific firefight he survived. These dreams are often related to trauma and replay unprocessed or avoided

memory content. For some people going through trauma, focused therapy helps with these nightmares. But for others, the nightmares may persist, even after a successful course of trauma treatment. That is, the nightmares can seem to take on a life of their own. This is how we would diagnose and treat nightmare disorder.

Sarah has idiopathic nightmares, as the content is not replaying any lived experiences. Toni's nightmares replay similar lived experiences from her work as a nurse, but blend in her grandmother (who has never been her patient).

What category best describes your most common nightmare? (Circle one.)

Idiopathic   **Symbolic**   **Replicative**   **I have more than one type**

Nightmares come from the part of our brain largely responsible for visual stimuli. The thoughts we have during the day, or in some cases avoid having, can also be related to nightmares. The part of our brain largely responsible for managing thoughts is the prefrontal cortex. This part of our brain is usually able to give feedback to the strong emotion centers and the visual cortex when we are awake. This feedback helps to regulate (or keep in check) the types of thoughts and images that we have. When we are asleep, the prefrontal cortex is far less active and far less able to give feedback to the emotional and visual centers of our brain. In addition, content that we're worried about, such as the strong emotions we feel, or anxiety and stressors that we may have gone to bed with, cannot be processed as well.

The prefrontal cortex is the logical, rational part of our brain. When it's offline, the visual cortex uses images to represent these unhelpful thoughts. For example, if you were having the thought, *I can't control anything that happens to me,* while awake, you may be able to rationalize that. You can reply, *I do have some control over things in my life, but I may not be able to control everything.* When you're asleep, the visual part of your brain may pull from images and memories to represent this lack of control, such as being pinned down in a firefight, being chased, or being unable to get to or reach something that could throw off a bad outcome. In addition, the emotional centers that are active in the night feed this with more fear, anxiety, apprehension, and distress—creating really upsetting pictures.

Think about it like a horror movie. The first time you watch a horror movie, you get startled. You may jump or even scream when the bad guy pops out. Your fight-or-flight system, the alarm system in your body, is going off intensely. If you watch that same movie a second time or even a third time, and certainly if you've seen it ten times, it does not seem as scary. Your body and brain start to recognize that this is not an immediate and real threat, saying, *This is not really happening to me right now*. Your prefrontal cortex is giving your body feedback to shut off the alarm.

However, the prefrontal cortex is not as able to do this while you sleep. So you need to help it by feeding your brain positive images, by reducing your overall anxiety levels, and by improving your sleep behaviors to stack the deck in your favor for when you sleep.

How can you get this visual center to stop giving you such disturbing imagery? Visualization gives the brain this new pathway to potentially go down. In this chapter, you'll do more work to strengthen that visual pathway. We will ask you to work on your nightmares while awake and rehearse them on a set schedule.

There are two paths you can take in this chapter. The two different, evidenced-based strategies will help address nightmares directly. Up to this point in the book, you have been using skills common across both proven treatments. At this choice point, you can consider which pathway is right for you. It may help to refer back to chapters 3 and 4 to review the information on exposure and rescription. Here are the differences in IRT and ERRT briefly.

IRT: We move forward with writing a new, pleasant dream in detail and ask you to rehearse this on a set schedule.

ERRT: We use a written exposure to the nightmare as a first step before rescripting the nightmare to a new dream. You would also rehearse the new dream on a set schedule.

How do you know which one is best for you? Both options work, regardless of your nightmares. But your co-authors often take different paths. Dr. Nadorff directs a community clinic that serves individuals with a wide range of disorders. While he sees patients with PTSD, it is not the focus of his generalist clinic. He most often starts with IRT, helping patients write a new dream first because it is easier but yet still works for the vast majority of people. However, if the nightmares do not get better with just using IRT, he is not afraid to add in exposure at that point. It's like trying less invasive interventions in other forms of medicine, starting with the less invasive IRT and moving from there.

Dr. Worley has worked across PTSD and behavioral sleep medicine specialty clinics primarily serving veterans. She usually sees patients with a history of trauma who have replicative nightmares about their trauma experiences. She most often has patients move through exposure and rescription, especially if patients have replicative nightmares that are very similar to their lived experience. However, we both emphasize patient choice in our work. The choice is yours. Both have strong research support, and we have included information if you start down one path and would like to change. We also include examples from Toni, Sarah, and John. Sarah is moving forward with IRT and focusing on rescripting a new dream only. Toni and John are both doing ERRT, exposure plus rescription. If you are undecided, here is more information about exposure.

Introducing Exposure

Exposure therapy is a well-researched and effective treatment for lots of different problems, including anxiety disorders, PTSD, and nightmares. It works by approaching feared content in a slow, systematic way to help retrain your body and brain to respond to cues that have become associated with something that causes you fear. As an example, some people develop a fear of dogs after a bad experience with a dog. Now certainly not all dogs are dangerous, but based on that bad experience, their body will respond with fear the next time they see a dog. This is how our body and our brain try to predict threats and keep us safe. However, this reaction can become overgeneralized, expanding to low-risk situations (seeing dogs on TV, in a park) and sometimes to all dogs, especially if someone avoids dogs. One way to help this person overcome their fear is through exposure.

Starting slowly with exposure to the feared stimulus (dogs), the person is allowed to experience the anxiety, and then notice the anxiety lessen over time. If they do this repeatedly, their brain and body will learn to tell the difference between a situation where a dog is a threat and where other dogs are low risk.

Many people would rather avoid dogs and that anxious feeling. Avoidance seems like a solution, but it starts to have a larger impact on our lives and the spaces where we can live our lives. For example, someone may stop going to a favorite park because there are dogs there, or maybe they don't go to a friend's house anymore because their Labrador will be home.

With nightmares, people learn avoidance by waking themselves up. Waking from the nightmare allows you to escape the situation and can become a habit. Some people also try to avoid sleep or delay sleep to avoid nightmares. None of these are effective long-term solutions, because human beings need sleep. Also, waking up from the nightmare (escaping) does not allow the brain to process the information. The brain gets stuck on nightmare content, which is why you may have the experience of returning to sleep and the nightmare. For trauma survivors, having the same nightmare repeated over and over again likely is another way of the brain trying to make sense of a senseless event and process the experience. Avoiding trauma content during the day may increase nightmares about that same content. The brain is trying to resolve the content, but it keeps getting stuck. We ultimately want you to be able to move past that stuck spot and sleep!

Scientists hypothesize that repeated exposure is an opportunity to learn to *habituate* to the feared stimulus, which is a big fancy word for anxiety reducing on its own in relation to the feared stimulus (Benito and Walther 2015). Recent research suggests that *inhibitory learning* may be a bigger cause of change in exposure therapy. Inhibitory learning is the idea that creating new information, and new learning about particular events, helps weaken older associations and thereby reduces the fear response (Sewart and Craske 2020). Regardless of how it works, we know that exposure therapy works and has benefitted many who have experienced traumas.

Exposure to the nightmare content does three things:

- Decreases the strength of the association between the nightmare content and immediate threat (through new learning)

- Increases your control over the content because you access it while awake and more able to recognize that it cannot harm you

- Decreases the physiological (body) reaction to nightmare content through habituation

Let's take a moment to address a concern that we often see in trauma survivors. Some trauma survivors believe that while the nightmare is distressing, if they stop having it, it means something negative. For example: *If I don't continue to dream about my friend's death, it means their service didn't matter, or other people will forget them if I don't continue to suffer.* While we won't talk much about these thoughts here, if you want to work on them, you will have that opportunity in chapter 11 on cognitive restructuring.

Pause to think about what your nightmares really mean to you. Is that meaning helpful or realistic in your life today?

_____

_____

_____

If you are grieving, or have lost loved ones, it's unlikely you'll forget your loved ones just because you don't have nightmares. Further, getting rid of the nightmare may create opportunities to recall more of the positive memories, or other parts of your relationship, and honor the person in different way.

When Is Exposure Not Recommended?

Exposure is a very valuable tool for treating nightmares and other disorders, but it is not the right fit for everyone. As you likely guessed, being exposed to something that is frightening to you, or a bad memory of something that happened in the past, can be disturbing and unpleasant. For this reason, if you are making good progress using imagery and improving your sleep skills, exposure may not be necessary. Likewise, exposure is commonly not needed for symbolic or idiopathic nightmares.

However, if you are not happy with your results from just using imagery and changing your sleep behaviors, then exposure may be a very good fit for you.

What are some of the benefits of exposure for you?

_____

_____

What are some of the drawbacks of exposure for you?

_____

_____

Are you thinking about trying exposure now? Why or why not?

_____
_____
_____
_____
_____

If you are, you can skip to the exposure section of this chapter. If you are not, let's introduce how to write your new dream.

Scripting a New Dream

If you could choose anything to dream about, what would you like to dream? This can be as creative as you would like. It can include important people, cultural elements, or a favorite vacation spot. The choices are many. The most important part is to create this new dream in great detail, paying attention to visual and sensory elements. The visual and emotional centers of your brain are most active at night. We will work on writing a dream you would like to have, and then practice will be important. Take a few minutes to brainstorm ideas of what you would like to dream about:

_____
_____
_____
_____
_____
_____

Before we work on writing your new dream in detail, let's look at Sarah's example. Sarah had the following nightmare.

I hear what sounds like my bedroom door opening, and I hear what I think may be some soft, careful footsteps coming toward me. I hear little creaks, not sure if it is just the sound of the house settling or my cat moving upstairs, or an intruder just feet away from me. I feel frozen with fear, trying not to move but also trying to keep my breathing as normal as possible to seem asleep. Finally, there is one last creak and then a warm sensation that feels like someone's breath against the back of my neck. At this point I am shocked awake, with my heart racing, sweating, and breathing very quickly. I turn on all the lights and do a pass to check the entire house, ensuring that no one is there and all the doors remain locked.

Here is the new dream she chose to write for herself.

Although I've never been there in person, I love looking at photos and travel videos of the Maldives. Each room in these resorts is a small villa that stands just a few feet over the water's surface on pilings, with a balcony that juts further out into the ocean, and a private stairway heading directly into the ocean. The rooms are open on one side, so you have an unbelievable view of the crystal blue water and the sunset each night. For my new dream, I want to be sitting on the balcony watching the sunset. Once the sun has completely gone down, I want to lie down in the bed and go to sleep. I hear sounds, but only the ocean rolling back and forth softly beneath me as the waves come in and go out. I feel the ocean breeze circulate the air in the room, and I can smell saltwater in the air. I feel safe and secure, and all the sounds I hear put me more at ease. The temperature is perfect, in the low 80s, but feeling cooler with the swirling ocean air. Every now and again, there's a brief hint of mist as a new wave comes in.

Sarah changed her dream significantly to make it a dream she would like to have! That is the key: it should be a dream you want to have, not just a less-negative version of your nightmare. Often when people struggle, it's because they did not change the dream enough to something they would really enjoy!

Now it's your turn. In this space, work on writing a new dream in as much detail as possible. Include sights, sounds, smells, and as many images as you can.

_____
_____
_____
_____
_____
_____
_____

The new dream now needs to be practiced during the day. We recommend practicing two times per day. Try to picture the image, in as much detail as possible. One of these times should be close to bedtime, but not in bed. When can you practice?

_____

_____

Include your practice on your sleep and nightmare logs. See if you notice any differences in your sleep and nightmares. This is not something that works overnight, but practice makes a difference. You can now jump to the end of this chapter to learn more about what to expect with the new dream.

Practicing Exposure

Take a few minutes to think about the nightmare you have most frequently or is the most distressing. This can be difficult. We want you to focus on the worst nightmare (if you have multiple) because you'll get the most benefit from starting there. In fact, you might not need to rescript a second nightmare if you start with the worst. If you are unsure which nightmare is the worst, use the one that has been most frequent in the last week.

In the following section please write out your worst nightmare. We want you to write it out in as much detail as you can with sights, sounds, smells, thoughts, and images, similar to the level of detail we ask for in the visualization exercise. For most people this takes about 10 minutes. You can set a timer for yourself if that would be helpful.

Before you begin writing, please take a moment to rate your SUDS level (0 to 10 level of distress).

My SUDS level is: _____

Describe your nightmare in writing, in as much detail as possible. Include the sounds, sights, smells, and tastes, thoughts you were thinking, and emotions you were feeling. Start at the very beginning of your nightmare and describe it up to the moment when you usually wake up. (If you dream more than "one version" of this nightmare, describe the most common version or the most upsetting version.)

_____

_____

_____

_____

_____

_____

_____

How do you feel after having completed the written exposure? Take a moment to rate your SUDS level (0 to 10 level of distress).

My post-writing SUDS level is: _____

Now use one of the relaxation strategies you have been practicing over the last few weeks. This could be deep breathing, progressive muscle relaxation, or visualization. Do this for about five minutes.

How do you feel after having completed the relaxation exercise (0 to 10 level of distress)?

My post-relaxation SUDS level is: _____

Write about what you learned from completing this exercise.

_____

_____

_____

Did your SUDS level increase after writing? **Yes No** (Circle one.)

It can be distressing to think about this nightmare content! However, thinking about your nightmare during the daytime (while you are fully awake) may not be quite as distressing because your prefrontal cortex is fully on, able to help with regulating. You know it's not happening now. It may not feel quite as real as it does when you are asleep.

Did your SUDS level go down after using relaxation? **Yes No** (Circle one.)

You may be like many people and felt your distress level decrease. Consider using relaxation strategies after a nightmare to help bring down the distress you feel. Reducing post-nightmare anxiety reactions can help you to return to sleep.

So, what happened from the post-writing SUDS to the post-relaxation SUDS? Especially if you've been practicing the relaxation, you'll notice that as your SUDS went down, you were able to bring on a relaxation response. You have more power over your nightmare now. You also have a tool that can increase relaxation. Now that you have this tool, you may choose to use it post nightmares to help to ground and center yourself, to help your ability to process, and to give feedback to the visual center of the brain as it comes back online too!

Rescripting the Nightmare

You have two options for how you approach the rescription. In the first option, you can change the dream at any point—beginning, middle, end. Maybe instead of starting in a dark wood, you start in a familiar place. Or maybe that scary thing behind you when you stop to confront it is actually your childhood cat coming to greet you. This option likely works better for nightmares that are more symbolic than historic.

In the second option, the new dream remains the same at the start. Keep the start of the nightmare the same. Then you will use the same well-worn nightmare pathway, and then put a fork in the road. This way, your brain can take a new trail and change the ending. This can be more effective for people with trauma-related dreams that have been recurring for years and years. The brain has such a habit of going down this path that it's easier to change the ending than to try starting a whole new dream. If you're willing, go back to the most difficult part of the nightmare you just wrote. Find where things start to get intense or scary. Put a star there, because it's going to be part of the rescription you learn next.

Remember Toni? Her nightmares have a theme of helplessness as she's unable to take care of her patients at work as a nurse. She doesn't know how to respond in situations where there's a medical emergency. For Toni, her nightmare is almost always the same situation: someone "codes" on her floor in the hospital. The patient can change, including sometimes looking like family members or friends. Here is Toni's original nightmare.

> I'm sitting at the nurse's station, charting orders. I wear blue scrubs that are my favorite. It's about an hour before my shift is over. It smells like disinfectant, as always, and I'm thirsty. I hear a lot of beeping, as always. Then all of a sudden, I see Tanya run past. Then I hear more footsteps, and I know something is about to happen. My heart starts beating and I stand up. I see a gurney coming down the hallway. I hear a code being called on the overhead system. I look down the hallway

and see my grandma going past on the gurney. She looks pale. Her eyes are closed. My coworkers are yelling, "Get the crash cart!" I feel frozen, like my shoes are stuck to the floor. I know I should be running as they go into trauma bay one, but I can't move. My grandma looks so small and frail in the bed. I see my coworkers running around her, and I want to cry out, but I can't do anything.

When you work on rescripting the nightmare, you can use the first part of the original nightmare to start. Then when the nightmare becomes scary or intense (the place you starred), you can make changes. Think about nightmares as a well-worn pathway through the woods. Your brain knows how to have the nightmare—it's a familiar route. Changing your dream using the skills of rescription is like creating a new pathway in the woods. Some people find it helpful to start down the same path and then take the fork in the road to create a new path and a new dream.

Rescription is an evidence-based strategy for addressing nightmares. It puts you in control of the script for your night and your dreams. You choose what you dream about by setting an intention. It usually takes practice, and most people need to rehearse the dream while awake to see changes in the night. There is a group of people who experience lucid dreaming (more in chapter 10) and can change their dreams and nightmares as they happen. However, for most people the changes need to happen while awake, during the time that the prefrontal cortex is online.

Before you work on your rescription, let's look at Toni's. Toni identified the hot spot as the point where she sees her grandmother on the gurney. Here is her rescription.

I'm sitting at the nurse's station, charting orders. I wear blue scrubs because they're my favorite. It's about an hour before my shift is over. It smells like disinfectant, as always, and I'm thirsty. I hear a lot of beeping, as always. Then all of a sudden, I see Tanya run past. Then I hear more footsteps, and I know something is about to happen. My heart starts beating and I stand up. I see a gurney coming down the hallway, and hear a code being called on the overhead system. I look down the hallway and see a young man going past on the gurney. He is awake and looks panicked. My coworkers are yelling, "Get the crash cart!" I move toward the room and take my position beside the bed. The physician is giving orders, and I work on moving smoothly and quickly, as part of the team. My adrenaline is pumping, and I use it to my advantage. We are able to stabilize the young man. From across the bed, Tanya nods at me. We've done this so many times before. I feel more confident. This is what we've trained for! We leave the room and as I return to the desk, I hear, "Good job, Toni!"

Now it's your turn. How would you like to change your nightmare? As you work on this new skill, remember: You are the author and director for this new story. The new dream should end in a way that is neutral, or more pleasant, than your original nightmare. You can choose what to dream and can change any aspect of the dream (where you are, who is there, and so on). Be creative here! Some like to add elements of fantasy, like giving themselves superpowers. Some add lighting or change the threat to something unthreatening. You can make any changes you want as long as you can represent them visually. Remember to include as many details as possible!

Rewrite your nightmare into a new dream with as much detail as possible. Include the sounds, sights, smells, and tastes, thoughts, and emotions you want to feel. Start at the very beginning of your nightmare, and change it at the moment when it usually becomes upsetting. At the end, *this should be a dream you would want to have*, not just a less negative dream.

Congratulations. You have taken another step on your recovery journey. Rewriting the nightmare one time during the day will not automatically change what happens at night. What will change your experience overnight is practice, so reread this new dream every day, two times a day, for the next week. It's important to practice reading this dream while engaging all your senses. Nightmares come from a part of the brain that is visual and emotional, so when you read through this new dream script, picture it in your mind.

Think about when you can practice. When can you find ten minutes during the day and ten minutes before bedtime to practice?

During the daytime, I will practice: _____

Before bedtime, I will practice: _____

Track this on your sleep diary. In the next week, you might notice you still have your target nightmare, which is typical. Or you could have the new dream. Often, people have a blend of the target nightmare and the new dream. Others report fewer dreams and nightmares because they are sleeping through the night and not waking up as much. All these are signs of progress. The most important thing is being consistent in your practice.

CHAPTER 9

Sleep Restriction and Stimulus Control

Did you know that if you sleep through a dream and do not have an awakening, you won't recall having the dream? We dream every night, but we will not remember those dreams unless they were interrupted or somehow led us to awaken. As a result, one way to help reduce your nightmares is to stay asleep. Two valuable tools come from cognitive behavioral therapy for insomnia (CBT-I): sleep restriction and stimulus control. They both have strong empirical support for helping you fall asleep on time and stay asleep. If you have trouble initiating sleep, or being awake in the middle of the night, this is the chapter for you.

Introduction to Stimulus Control

Do you always engage in some behavior in a certain spot or under certain conditions—and you feel pulled to engage in that behavior going forward? I experience this when I want to drive to my daughter's school over the summer, even though I do not need to drop her off. Or when I sit in my seat by the television, I feel a craving for snacks. These associations are built up over time and can modify our behavior, whether we realize it or not. The same can happen with sleep! Certain places or pieces of furniture can become associated with sleeping, or more problematically, not sleeping.

If you struggle with insomnia, you may find that your bed is actually associated with being awake and not being asleep. Even though you sleep in the bed every night, you may lie in bed hoping to fall asleep, trying to fall asleep, but not falling asleep. All that time (sometimes hours upon hours), spent associating bed with being awake, not with being asleep.

Do you find that you sleep better when not at home, maybe in a hotel? While this could be due to different reasons (like having an old bed that needs to be replaced, or the hotel has less stimuli that wake you up), it can indicate that you have a learned association between bed and wakefulness. If you go to bed feeling dead tired, but as soon as your head hits the pillow you feel wide awake, this is also a sign that you may be having trouble with a learned association. The good news is, because this is learned, you can also unlearn this behavior! More on this later in this chapter.

Introduction to Sleep Restriction

Have you ever tried to sleep in, or take a nap on a weekend, and find that no matter what you do you just cannot fall asleep? Why is this? The answer, as you will likely remember from chapter 5, is your homeostatic sleep drive. Simply put, there is only so much sleep your body can generate, much like you can only eat so much and sometimes there's no space for dessert. Recall the gas tank metaphor. Ideally, you want your fuel to be all the way at empty when you go to bed. Being empty is associated with having the highest sleep pressure, or sleep drive. This is how your body works with you to go to sleep. Then, you want to be all the way full in the morning.

However, what happens when you go to bed, and you still have a quarter tank of gas? Well, one of two things. You may not have enough sleep pressure to fall asleep, and this results in being awake until your gas is depleted enough to finally go to sleep. Or you end up filling up your gas tank too early, and this leads to waking up in the middle of the night or too early in the morning.

How does this system get off-kilter like this? It often happens through minor compensatory behaviors that make sense on the surface but end up leading to problems. For instance, when you nap, you not only stop burning gas, but you actually add some to your tank. Likewise, if you sleep in, you can start burning gas too late in the day. Either of these can lead to having a quarter tank left at bedtime.

In sleep restriction, sometimes now better described as *sleep retraining*, you determine how much sleep you can generate. Then you limit your time in bed to the amount of sleep you can generate. This ensures you are only in bed for as much time as you can generate sleep for, and you are not in bed trying to get more sleep when your gas tank is all the way full already.

Implementation

So how do you implement these strategies in your sleep schedule? First, a few words of caution. It's possible that your sleep may get worse in the short term, but it will improve your sleep in the coming days to weeks! If you have a history of seizures or have been diagnosed with bipolar disorder, you should not do sleep restriction. It can worsen both of those disorders.

To do sleep restriction safely, you need to ensure that you do not reduce the amount of sleep you are getting. If you want to try it, let's get started with sleep restriction. Otherwise, skip this part.

The Sleep Diary

This treatment is very data-driven, so as we did in earlier chapters, you will use your sleep diary to guide this process. You're going to calculate a few key metrics to guide your work.

Time in bed: This is the amount of time between when you first laid down to bed (number 1 on the sleep diary) to the time you got out of bed in the morning (number 7 on the sleep diary). This can be tricky to calculate if you went to bed before midnight, so figure out how long before midnight you went to bed. Then add that to when you got out of bed. For instance, if you went to bed at ten o'clock p.m. and got out of bed at six o'clock a.m., you would calculate two hours between when you went to bed and midnight. Then adding that to six hours. Your *time in bed* totals eight hours.

Total sleep time: As it sounds, this is how much time you slept during the night. This one is a bit trickier to calculate, so let's talk through it! The easiest way to calculate it is to start with the time that you wanted to sleep and then subtract the time that you were not able to sleep. For instance, let's say you were hoping to sleep starting at ten o'clock p.m. (in this case, number 2 on the sleep diary, as this can be different than when you got into bed). You woke up for the last time in the morning (number 6 on the sleep diary, let's say 5:30 a.m.). Doing the math as we did for your *time in bed*, we would get seven hours, thirty minutes. However, you need to account for the time it took to fall asleep and any time you were awake during the night. So subtract the time in row 3 (how long it took you to fall asleep) and row 5 (how long your total awakenings lasted). Let's say it took you thirty minutes to fall asleep, and then you were awake in the middle of the night for thirty more minutes. Subtract these values from the sleep time you calculated earlier. Here's the equation: 7 hours, 30 minutes – 30 minutes – 30 minutes = 6 hours, 30 minutes. Your *total sleep time* was six hours and thirty minutes.

Sleep efficiency: Last, calculate your sleep efficiency—the proportion of time that you are actually sleeping when in bed. To do this, take your *total sleep time* and divide it by *your time in bed*. For this example, divide six hours, thirty minutes by eight hours. The easiest way to do this is to convert the time spans to minutes. Multiply the hours by sixty. Then add the minutes. In our example, you had a total sleep time of six hours, which when converted to minutes, is 360 minutes. Then add in the thirty additional minutes, which leaves you with a total sleep time of 390 minutes. Likewise, do this for time in bed—multiplying eight hours by sixty, which equals 480 minutes. Thus, we divide 390 by 480 to get a *sleep efficiency* of 81.25 percent.

Sleep opportunity: Now that you know how to calculate some key variables, you'll need to do it for every day, over the last week, that you recorded in your sleep diary. This will help you know your *average total sleep time* over the course of a week. It's how much sleep you can generate. Let's say over the course of the week, you averaged seven hours and thirty minutes of sleep. We add thirty minutes to this total because research shows we tend to underestimate how much we actually sleep (Manconi et al. 2010). You end up with eight hours. This is how much *sleep opportunity* you should allow when setting your sleep schedule.

Sleep prescription: You want to allow for eight hours of sleep opportunity, so you need to set a sleep prescription. This is the time you go to bed and wake up every day, even on weekends. This consistency is important, at least for the short term, to help get your body get used to when it should be asleep and when it should be awake. The first step is to determine what time you need to be up by for your earliest day. If there is one day in the week you need to wake up by six o'clock a.m. for example, then you would set your wake time to six o'clock a.m. every day. From there, calculate your *sleep prescription* by working backward to determine that the bedtime you need to have is ten o'clock p.m. Then you'll allow for eight hours of *sleep opportunity*.

Tracking and refining: Once you have the sleep prescription set, the next step is to try it out for a week. During this time, it's important to complete the sleep log so you can use the data to determine next steps. Specifically, your *sleep efficiency* is going to be the data point you use. At the end of each week, calculate your sleep efficiency to determine whether it's 85 percent or higher. If it is, you can move your bedtime earlier by fifteen minutes. In the example, you'd move to a 9:45 p.m. bedtime. You can keep doing this until either: you're satisfied with the amount of sleep you're getting; or your sleep efficiency is below 85 percent, indicating that you are not able to generate enough sleep to fill your sleep opportunity. If the latter happens, move your bedtime fifteen minutes later, to the last prescription where you had at least 85 percent sleep efficiency. Then lock it in!

While you're working on changing your sleep schedule, it's a good time to start implementing stimulus control strategies. You'll work to make your bed and bedroom associated with being asleep and not with being awake. To do this, ensure that the times you are in the bed (and ideally, the broader bedroom) are when you're sleeping. Restrict the bed and bedroom to sleep and sexual activity only. Avoid watching television, being on your phone, reading, or even being in bed if you are not asleep.

How does this work? Go to bed at your bedtime and lie down for sleep. If you fall asleep, great! However, if fifteen minutes pass (approximately, do not stare at a clock as that could keep you up) or it has been long enough that you are agitated about not falling asleep, go ahead and get out of bed. If possible, even leave the bedroom. During this time, do something enjoyable but not too activating. Watching television or reading a print book (not on a tablet or phone) are both good candidates. Avoid laptops, phones, and tablets because they emit blue light, which signals your brain that it's time to be awake. Don't exercise or do things that are activating during this time, as the goal is to be able to return to bed as soon as possible.

Once you feel tired, go back to bed and try to go to sleep again with the same rules. Hopefully you go to sleep. But if you do not, are agitated that you have not fallen asleep, or about fifteen minutes have passed, go ahead and once again get out of bed. Return to the activity you were doing beforehand. You might feel like a yo-yo for a few nights, going back and forth, to and from the bedroom. But this is how you'll build an association between bed and sleep. As time goes on, this association will build. It will get easier and easier, and you will find that you rarely need to leave the bed.

Troubleshooting Your Implementation

We will be honest, implementing sleep restriction and stimulus control is among the hardest treatments in behavioral sleep medicine. So you may run into some challenges or concerns. Because of that, here are the primary challenges and concerns that come up in our practice. We have found the following ways to work around, or manage, them as best as possible.

Not getting enough sleep: One concern is about getting enough sleep! You just set a sleep schedule that only provides enough sleep opportunity for the sleep you can generate. But if you're getting up and leaving the bedroom, it may mean that you don't maximize the amount of sleep you could get. It is absolutely likely that you will sleep a bit worse for a night or two. This is why one of our favorite mantras is "If not tonight, then tomorrow." If you do not get enough sleep tonight, it will increase your sleep debt and sleep drive for tomorrow night. Your odds that tomorrow's sleep will be better, more consolidated and restful, increase.

Staying up later: It's not uncommon for your new sleep schedule to require you to stay up far later than you are used to. This makes sense, because in sleep restriction you're reducing your sleep opportunity, so it's expected that there will be less time in bed. Given this, you may need to go to bed several hours later than you're used to! So how do you stay up that late? A lot of the advice still applies: Do activities that are not too activating but that you enjoy. Reading, watching television, even being on the computer, phone, or tablet during this time will keep you awake enough. Exercising is less ideal, because it's too activating this close to bed. There are many other options. Try to use the time to do something you've been wanting to do but have not had the time to get to. Then you get the two-for-one benefit of staying up later and also accomplishing something that has been on your list for a while.

Leaving the bed is impossible: You may not able to leave the bedroom, or even the bed. College students, for instance, often live in dorms where leaving the bedroom really isn't possible. Those with physical limitations may be unable to leave the bed without assistance. In these cases, do the best you can. A college student can limit the bed to sleep and sexual activity, even if the rest of the bedroom cannot be used exclusively for those activities. If you are unable to leave the bed, try splitting the bed in half, with one half being a sleep side and the other being an awake side. This way, if you have not fallen asleep fast enough, you can roll over to the awake side. We don't recommend that strategy if you are able to get out of the bed, but if you are unable, it is a viable strategy.

We know these are challenging skills, but if you are struggling with insomnia, they truly are game changers. It's important to pick the right time to implement them, as you may not sleep as well for a few days to a week. But once you get used to the new setup, and your body starts associating your bed with being asleep and not fighting you all night, you will see that these strategies are investments that pay dividends for years to come!

CHAPTER 10

Lucid Dreaming and Lucidity Checks

THE NIGHTMARE & SLEEP DISORDER TOOLKIT

So far, we've taught you the basics of sleep and strategies you can apply during the day, while you're awake, to change your bad dreams and nightmares. You can also change your nightmare *while you are having it* through lucid dreaming. Have you ever thought, *What if I could take control of my dream? Then I would finally be able to manage these bad dreams and get a handle on them.* You are not alone. Lucid dreams have fascinated both scientists and laypeople for a very long time. Lucid dreaming happens when you become aware of the fact that you are asleep *while* you are having a dream. There are three stages of lucidity:

1. **Awareness:** You become aware that you are asleep and dreaming, but you are not able to change things about the dream.

2. **Control of self:** You are able to guide your own behavior and actions, but you do not have power over others or the environment.

3. **Control of self and environment:** You not only are aware that you are asleep, and have control of yourself, but you also have control over the environment. You could change where you are, manifest people to be a part of the dream, and direct the action!

Have you ever experienced one or all of these stages?

If yes, think about a dream or nightmare where you had awareness. What were you able to control?

_____

_____

_____

_____

_____

If not, you can work on developing this skill. While some people are more likely to have lucid dreams, anyone can cultivate this skill through practice.

You can likely immediately see why lucid dreams have the potential to help people who suffer from nightmares. Indeed, while the literature on it isn't as rich as the research supporting imagery rescripting, a recent systematic review of lucid dreaming research found encouraging results in improving nightmares through lucid dreaming therapy (Ouchene, El Habchi, Demina, Petit, and Trojak 2023).

Are you ready to take control of your dreams? If so, continue reading for empirically supported strategies to induce lucidity and start on this journey of becoming an active participant in your dreams!

Reality Testing and Dreams

You have undoubtedly heard people say, "Let me pinch myself," to ensure an experience is real and not a dream. In many ways, reality testing is the opposite of this principle—you're going to be testing to ensure that you are asleep and not awake. This sounds simple at first, but that's because pinching ourselves while awake is quite simple and under our control. How do we do this while asleep? By doing it multiple times during the day!

When you think about it, there are everyday things you do that make it into your dreams. Have you had dreams about forgetting your locker combination, or even forgetting to get dressed? These activities (dressing, opening a locker) are things you did, or still do, on a daily basis. Because of this, they have worked their way into your dreams. In the same way, you can work lucidity checks into your dreams by mindfully building them into your day.

What are these lucidity checks like? Different checks work differently for each person. I've heard numerous stories across the years about what checks work, so here are some of my favorite checking methods. However, you do not have to do all of these, or you can try others. The main purpose is for the check to be something you can easily do several times during your day. Here are some examples of actions that can help you recognize you are in a dream. If you cannot complete these tasks, you will know you are not awake.

- Push on solid objects. Test reality by pushing on things! Objects we can push are not solid in dreams.

- Put your fingers on your palm. If you put your fingers on your palm and push down while dreaming, you will very often be able to push right through your hand.

- Put your hand on a table. If you are near a table and push down, similarly, when dreaming your hand will sink right through the table.

- Turn on or off lights. Lights do not typically work the same in our dreams as they do in real life. As long as your light is functional and the power is on, if you flip a switch the lights are likely to come on (or go off) in the room. However, when you flip a switch in dreams, typically nothing happens!

- Open a door. In dreams, you can twist the handle on a door and nothing happens. Or if you lock or unlock the door, there will be no change when you try to open it.

- Check the time. Numbers commonly act differently in dreams! If you look at a clock to see the time, look away, and then look back at the clock, chances are you will see a very different time. Likewise, page numbers in a book or numbers in a newspaper can be used the same way. Performing simple math can also be an option, as in a dream you likely cannot complete an equation.

- Read a book. In dreams, we cannot just sit and read.

These are just a few strategies that have been used successfully to induce lucidity. There are many others. What strategy would you like to try for lucidity checks?

_____

_____

_____

Now that you have identified a strategy, let's talk about the best way to practice it. The more you practice lucidity checks, the more likely they will start appearing in your dreams. Some find that setting a timer for one to two hours is a good way to remember to do your brief lucidity checks throughout the day. This is especially helpful if you are pushing an object, like your hand or a table. Another strategy is, when you pass by a door, try locking and unlocking the door to see if it changes whether or not it opens. Or if you pass a light, turn the switch a few times to make sure that the light turns on and off. (Though perhaps do not use these strategies when others are in the room.) Regardless, it is important to be regular, practicing whatever your lucidity check of choice is, several times per day. This will help them enter your dreams, and that is where the real fun begins!

There are two primary strategies for inducing lucid dreaming: MILD and reality testing. The MILD strategy includes reality testing, and also includes some additional techniques.

The MILD Strategy of Inducing Lucid Dreams

MILD stands for the *mnemonic induction of lucid dreams*. It was developed by well-known dream researcher Dr. Stephen LaBerge. Essentially, the MILD technique helps set your intention for having lucid dreams and arranges the stage so you are in the best position to have them.

In addition to the reality checks, MILD includes *lucidity affirmations* to help encourage your mind to allow you to have lucid dreams. These should be simple, easy-to-follow mantras such as, *I will have lucid dreams tonight*, or, *I will be in control of my dreams tonight*. Repeat these mantras either aloud or in your mind over and over, really focusing on them, setting your intention toward having lucid dreams. This is best done shortly before going to sleep so the mantra is one of the last thoughts you have before drifting off.

MILD includes some visualization like we did in chapter 7, but it has a different focus and intention. In chapters 7 and 8, we discussed how to rescript a dream and use imagery with the new dream to introduce that content to the brain. As we will discuss, the visualization differs in MILD from the visualization in chapter 7 in several key ways:

- When the visualization occurs
- What you visualize
- The intention behind the visualization

Timing is important in the MILD strategy, as you practice right before you drift off to sleep. You should practice your mantra and then the visualization of the desired vivid dream. This differs from the nightmare rescription technique, which is practiced during the day.

What you visualize is different also. MILD recommends that you visualize a recent vivid dream (non-nightmare) that you have had. If you do not have one you can visualize, you can visualize a dreamlike scenario you would like to have. As you did in chapter 7, include as much detail as possible, looking for potential signs that it's a dream through identifying things that happen that would not happen in real life. The intention behind this is different.

In chapter 7, the focus was on changing your dream so you have a new, nonthreatening dream. In MILD, the goals are to increase the likelihood of moving into that dream as you fall asleep, prime yourself to be able to find those dream signs, become lucid that you are asleep, and then be set up to start changing the dream.

MILD is a nice addition to reality testing, as it helps with setting your intention clearly before you go to bed and then priming your brain for the dream you want to have.

Which strategies do you want to try?

_____

_____

_____

Develop a Customized Lucid Dreaming Practice

Practice is absolutely essential for most nightmare treatments to work, and lucid dreaming is no different. Because of this, it's important to develop a practice plan that is feasible.

Which strategies did you select? Once you have decided, think through a way to practice them at least six times each day. Each session should take no more than a minute or two at most, so it's easy to fit into your day. Do you want to set alarms on your phone to remind yourself to do the practice, or start practicing every time you do something like unlock a door or turn on a light? Whatever it is, write down your plan below. Are you confident that you will be able to do it multiple times per day every day?

_____

_____

_____

Now that you have your reality testing set, it's a good time to decide whether you want to build in the MILD strategy as well. This practice is up to you—you are in control! If you are doing the reality testing, you are hitting the minimum required practice, so adding in MILD is for extra credit. It further increases the odds of success.

How does MILD fit with your bedtime routine? Do you feel like you can incorporate it into your routine as-is, or would it require going to bed about ten to fifteen minutes earlier? Are there any aspects that you would rather not practice?

_____

_____

_____

_____

_____

_____

While many people can learn to lucid dream, unfortunately not everyone is able to, and it is a struggle for some to learn these skills. If you are not having luck, please do not lose hope. It takes time. Just like any skill, the more you practice the better you get. The effects of the reality testing also build upon themselves over time. Think about it: we dream about forgetting our locker combination, or driving to work, but those were things happening every day. Unless they were particularly notable or traumatic, how often do you dream about things that happened just once or twice? Probably never, right? This is the same way—the more you practice, and do so over time, the more likely it is to work into your dream.

Once you obtain lucidity, you may struggle with being able to harness it. As we discussed earlier, there are three levels of lucidity: being aware that you are dreaming, being able to change your own behavior, and being able to influence others and settings. You may find that you become lucid in your dream but are stuck at the first stage for a while. That's alright; it's a huge accomplishment just to obtain lucidity, so first of all congratulate yourself for reaching that milestone! As you become lucid during your dreams more and more, continue practicing within the dream. First, become able to affect what you do, and as you obtain this, then try to move on to others. As with all the skills, it takes time but is well worth it.

Applying Lucidity to Nightmares

Once you obtain lucidity and are able to change things in your dream, do not hesitate to do so! If you are having a nightmare and are lucid, that is great, that is what you have been working up to and training for. Don't be afraid of trying something different. If it is a nightmare of a dog that is always chasing you, don't hesitate to try standing your ground to see if you get a different outcome. Once you reach the third stage, where you can affect the environment, then you can put a fence between you and the dog or add in other defenses. Remember, it is a dream. You can do nearly anything, so allow yourself to be creative! Lucid dreaming allows you to take control over your dreams, so do not hold back. With control over your dreams comes the power you need to have the dreams you want to have and transform the night!

CHAPTER 11

Cognitive Restructuring

Take a few minutes to think about how you think about your sleep. That is, what are you telling yourself about your sleep? Likely these thoughts are automatic and happen without you being fully aware of them. Common times to have automatic negative thoughts about sleep are when you aren't sleeping well. Maybe when you're having difficulty falling asleep, maybe when you wake up from a nightmare, or when you find that you wake up in the morning too early. Some people also notice they have negative automatic thoughts about sleep throughout the day. These negative thoughts can worsen sleep problems, mood, and prolong awakenings. This can further the nightmare cycle and impact insomnia or other mental health conditions. To see if this chapter might be helpful for you, see if any of these thoughts fit for you now, or in the past. (Check all that apply.)

- [ ] If I fall asleep now, I can still get X hours
- [ ] I won't be able to sleep unless I… (take sleeping pills, drink alcohol, and so on)
- [ ] If I stop having my nightmares, I'm going to forget my friend
- [ ] If I stop having my nightmare, I might miss important cues (the dream is warning me)
- [ ] If I sleep longer than two hours, I'm in danger (I need to get up and check)
- [ ] I have no control over my sleep
- [ ] I have no control over my nightmare
- [ ] I can never be a healthy sleeper
- [ ] My health is damaged because of my sleep
- [ ] I need eight hours to be able to function the next day
- [ ] I know I'm going to have a nightmare tonight

If any or many of these thoughts seem familiar, it is likely worth spending some time with this chapter on cognitive restructuring. Earlier in this workbook, we said the part of your brain that deals with thoughts is not as active during sleep. So why are we discussing thoughts? Thoughts during the day certainly impact sleep. Many people who struggle with their sleep start to predict that their bad sleep is going to persist *or* get worse. Addressing the thoughts you have about your sleep is another way to interrupt the nightmare cycle. Some people who struggle with negative thoughts due to depression or anxiety may notice a change in thoughts or in sleep when their other mental health symptoms are worse. Addressing negative thoughts about sleep can also help with managing increasing symptoms for other mental health concerns.

Because sleep problems are a 24-hour problem, we ask you to pay attention throughout the day and notice thoughts you have about your sleep. Write down a few notes about thoughts that come up for you at different times. You may fill this out now and then monitor your thoughts over the next week to add later.

Bedtime thoughts: _____

_____

_____

_____

_____

Thoughts during middle-of-the-night awakenings: _____

_____

_____

_____

_____

Thoughts upon waking up in the morning: _____

_____

_____

_____

_____

Daytime thoughts: _____
_____
_____
_____
_____

In working with patients with both insomnia and nightmares across our careers, we have found that people often relate to the bedtime thoughts most. Is this a familiar scenario?

You're falling asleep on the couch watching television. You go to bed and are suddenly wide awake! You start feeling irritable, anxious, and then the thoughts start: *I'm never going to fall asleep. How many nightmares am I going to have tonight? Here we go again. This is seriously damaging my health. No way, I'm not going to be ready for my presentation at work tomorrow. I'm going to get fired!*

These anxious thoughts are not only annoying, but they are also feeding the nightmare cycle. Increased anxious thoughts at bedtime can increase nightmare risk in a few ways.

Anxious Feelings at Bedtime May Delay Sleep Onset

One of the theories for why insomnia persists after bad sleep in some people is called *conditioned arousal.* This means people start to get stressed out when they get into the bed because they're telling themselves something bad is going to happen. Sometimes this conditioned arousal is a result of classical conditioning. In chapter 9, we shared why stimulus control is really important. What you do in the bed gets paired with the bed and your brain gets trained to do those things. You want to pair the bed with sleep, but in some instances the more you lie awake in bed, the more you have negative thoughts. If you've ever had negative thoughts while in bed, you may want to work on *cognitive restructuring*—or changing your thinking about sleep. Delaying sleep onset pulls you out of rhythm with the sleep your body needs and the timing of that sleep. We are trying to keep your sleep pattern as consistent as possible.

If you have a history of trauma, conditioned arousal may extend beyond the bed. You may have hyperarousal symptoms, in which your nervous system goes into overdrive trying to find and predict threats. The body has a natural reaction called *fight or flight* that should turn on when we are in danger. However, with a history of trauma, this system is often overactive. This system can be thought of like a light switch, where being alert is the "on" and relaxation (needed for sleep) is the "off." Light switches cannot be in both the off and on position at the same time. Hyperarousal stays on, blocking your body's natural sleep drive. Additionally, the feelings associated with this state can lead to safety behaviors, such as checking locks and doors, sleeping with the light on, sleeping with weapons, and so on. All this provides feedback to the body that you need to stay alert. If your trauma happened at night, in a bed, just the idea of being asleep and more vulnerable can add layers to the stress. People with nightmares often make predictions about having nightmares! Or have anxious thoughts about safety.

Anxious Thoughts at Bedtime Can Increase Nightmares

Remember the mood matching theory we talked about in chapter 6? The emotions you feel at bedtime may get picked up by the brain. It then pulls images or stories to match those emotions. When you go to bed anxious or fearful, you are more likely to have nightmares. Providing the brain with calmer emotions and thoughts at bedtime reduces the likelihood of that imagery. This is another reason why we taught you relaxation in chapter 6 and visualization in chapter 7.

How to Work with Negative Thoughts About Sleep

Let's start looking at your thoughts about sleep and test them out and see how realistic or helpful they may be. If you've ever worked with a therapist on cognitive behavioral therapy interventions, you may have learned similar skills. If not, don't worry! This is a skill we can work on together in this workbook.

A common way we address unhelpful thoughts in treatment for sleep, anxiety, depression, and trauma is to have people pay attention to their thoughts, and then start to examine those thoughts in a very purposeful way. Sometimes we also use behavioral experiments to consider thoughts about sleep. Here's a common thought you may notice when you are in bed awake.

I won't be able to function without eight hours of sleep.

Does this thought, or some version of it, sound familiar? Certainly, this is a popular myth that everyone needs eight hours of sleep. In tracking your sleep across this book, you have likely found the amount of sleep where you feel your best. If you've made it this far in life, you've also likely had times where you have functioned on less than eight hours. Maybe it wasn't your best day, but you likely were not completely unable to function. This thought may not be completely true, and it certainly isn't helping you fall or stay asleep. So how do negative thoughts like this one impact your sleep? Negative thoughts impact sleep in three possible ways:

- Create negative emotions (like anxiety, frustration, fear, or anger)
- Increase nightmare risk through mood matching, which makes your brain reach for images that match negative emotions at bedtime
- Worsen sleep and create more distress the next day, which continues the cycle of nightmares with more broken sleep and daytime distress

If these things are happening, you are likely more aware of when things go wrong. Being primed to notice worse functioning further supports, or feeds, the negative thought. Now, we're not going to argue that you're probably at peak functioning on four hours of sleep! Very few people can or will be able to sustain that. But it's likely you have been able function on less-then-ideal sleep for a while. It also means you are looking for ways to change. If you can choose how to interact with your thoughts, you may be able to promote healthier sleep and recovery from the nightmare cycle.

Toni identified some unhelpful thoughts interacting with her sleep. She identified the following thoughts and took some notes about how they made her feel. Using her sleep diary, she tracked when she was having more negative thoughts and noticed how they were linked to her sleep and nightmares that night.

Timing	Thoughts	Emotions
Bedtime	I know I'm going to have another nightmare.	Anxious
Waking from a nightmare	I have no control! I'm not safe anywhere. I will always have nightmares.	Fearful, frustrated
Woke at 5 a.m. when my alarm was set for 6:30 a.m.	I'm going to feel awful at work. I can't keep having these nightmares.	Irritated

Those are a lot of thoughts about sleep and nightmares, and they all seem to be producing negative emotions and sleeplessness for Toni. She noticed a connection between these thoughts and how long it took her to fall asleep. These thoughts happened more often on nights when she was distressed at bedtime, and they seemed to predict more nightmares. On those nights, she also had longer stretches of time awake after having nightmares where she worried about even more things.

What can be done about thoughts? These thoughts are likely automatic, and Tori certainly isn't trying to have these thoughts! To help Tori with cognitive restructuring, we asked her to stop and evaluate the thoughts during the day. She was asked to look over her notes and choose one thought to practice this new skill of cognitive restructuring on.

What Is Cognitive Restructuring?

Cognitive is another word for "thinking." Cognitions are the internal thoughts that you have about yourself, others, your sleep, and your functioning. Negative thoughts about sleep are common in people with sleep problems, but you may notice negative thoughts in other areas. One common thought we've already highlighted is, *If I don't sleep enough, I won't be able to function tomorrow.* Another common automatic negative thought we hear is, *I will never sleep well again.*

Restructuring is a way of breaking down thoughts and asking questions about them. Sometimes this involves becoming more aware of the thoughts and when they are happening. You can then use skills to test out the thoughts or change them to be more helpful or more realistic.

We are not trying to say your thoughts are not real! We believe you are having problems with sleep and nightmares that impact your daytime functioning. However, many people become focused on the negative thoughts and those thoughts fuel the sleep problems they already have. Negative thoughts can often become more extreme over time and add to the nightmare cycle. This happens through *selective attention*. It's normal to look for evidence to support existing beliefs or experiences—and ignore or discount other information. This is not unique to sleep problems, but when you have sleep problems it's often easier to recall sleepless nights and nightmares. Sometimes improvements are discounted, seen as exceptions, or just harder to recall. This is one reason we have encouraged you to track your sleep in the sleep and nightmare logs. You may be good at remembering you felt bad or slept poorly but not recognize the changes that happen over time. This may be true especially early in this process when you still had more bad nights than good ones.

Most negative thoughts are not helpful, as they worsen mood. They also do not help you to change your behavior. Through cognitive restructuring, you'll pay attention to your thoughts about sleep and whether they are helpful or even supported by facts. There are facts to support your experience having sleep problems; however, these thoughts may not help your sleep and nightmares. Take a moment to reflect.

When has worrying about your sleep improved your sleep?

___

___

How have negative thoughts about sleep improved your nightmares?

___

___

It's likely you answered "never" and "they make nightmares worse." So let's try adding cognitive restructuring skills to your toolkit.

Finding Evidence for Your Case

One of the ways we can work on thoughts is to think about evidence for and against them. We like to use a trial metaphor, like in a court of law. Put this thought on trial. Let's use the thought, *I cannot function on less than eight hours of sleep.*

The sleep problem is the prosecution, and your recovery is the defense. The prosecution is loudly giving all kinds of evidence that supports your negative thought.

"Remember how tired you were?"

"See how you made those mistakes at work?"

"Remember how you snapped at your family?"

Those things may be true or partially true, but let's also let the defense talk! The "defense" is your recovery from nightmares. The defense gives you this evidence.

"You have still been able to go to work."

"You did well on that presentation."

"You still made it to your kid's soccer match."

"You showed up for a friend in an important conversation."

This is not to say that you should always be functioning on two hours of sleep! However, noticing that you can still function might help to reduce some of the nighttime anxiety and next day frustration and irritability.

If we take all these pieces of information together, we might come up with a more balanced thought like, *If I don't get eight hours, I may feel tired, but I can still do the important things in my life.*

Let's look at how Toni started working on some of her thoughts about sleep. Toni thought it would be easier to work on her early awakening thoughts. She chose this one because waking up in the middle of the night often was not the best time for her to start thinking. She worried that if she tried to change her thought in the middle of the night first, she might just stay up worrying. When Toni did this activity, it looked like this.

Thought	Feeling	Evidence For	Evidence Against
I'm going to feel awful at work!	Irritated	Some days I feel bad when I'm working.	There've been days I was okay. Sometimes it's more about who I work with than how much sleep I get.

Tori recognized that this is a thought that might sometimes be true, but it might not be true 100 percent of the time. She also recognized that there may be other things impacting her day besides her sleep. Over a week, she recognized:

- She usually had a good day working with her close friend, Tia.

- She worried less about her sleep on days when she was busy and felt confident in what she was doing.

- When she felt bad, it was not just caused by her sleep. She could point to a few times where things were not going right at work, but when she was able to resolve a problem or move to a different task, her mood usually improved.

After noticing these things, Toni began looking more for both sides of the argument that *I'm going to feel awful at work*. She also tried to avoid predicting how she would feel at work. Toni wondered if her thoughts were looking for evidence that she was feeling bad and only attributing it to her sleep.

After another week of tracking, Tori collected more information and was working on reviewing this information. She started working on a new thought to replace the older thought, *I'm going to feel awful at work*. First, she started talking back to the thought and listing the reasons why it was not 100 percent true. However, this was difficult and too much to do each time this thought came up. She drafted a few options for alternative thoughts to try during the week. They included:

- *I may not have slept well, but I can still be productive*

- *I have had worse nights of sleep and still been successful*

- *I'm still working on my sleep and on me*

- *This too shall pass*

She used these thoughts when the old thought popped up. And she started practicing these thoughts when she woke up. She put one in her phone as a reminder to help her practice. She particularly liked using this one first thing in the morning: *I'm still working on my sleep and on me.*

Toni also started to consider that there were things she could do first thing in the morning if she woke up early. She knew lying in bed worrying was not improving her sleep or attitude. She considered that waking up thirty minutes earlier might give her an opportunity to do things that would improve her daytime functioning. She brainstormed a list, including practicing yoga, taking more time with her morning coffee, or brushing and petting her dog. Tori planned an experiment to test out these new activities and this new thought: *Getting up earlier means I have time for myself.*

Thoughts About Nightmares

For trauma survivors, beliefs about the trauma and what it means to keep having reminders of it (through daytime thoughts or memories, and nightmares) can be important to consider. Here are some common thoughts about nightmares. Do any of these look familiar?

- *I'm being punished by these nightmares. I deserve to have them because I've done bad things.*

- *I need to learn from these nightmares.*

- *God, or my higher power, is trying to teach me something through these nightmares.*

- *If I can force myself not to think about the nightmare, I'll be less likely to have it.*

- *If I don't keep having the nightmare, I'll forget my friends.*

- *Having the nightmares keeps me aware of bad things that could happen, so I can prepare.*

John certainly didn't like having nightmares. However, he also worried that if he didn't have the nightmares, he might not remember his friends and he might be in danger. In some ways, John felt having the nightmares kept him safer. As much as he didn't want to have the nightmares, he also had some hesitation about getting rid of the nightmares. He noticed the thoughts about safety were somewhat better, based on the work he did in earlier chapters of this workbook. He was not sleeping with the lights on in his room anymore. He also was doing less checking of the house. John chose to work on this thought: *If I don't keep having the nightmare, I'll forget my friends.*

One of the ways John worked to address this thought was to consider times—other than nightmares—when he thought about his friends from Vietnam. He started to think he'd much rather remember positive experiences that he had with them, than to relive their injuries every night. He also thought about ways he could honor them without sacrificing his sleep. John took a few days to think about this. He realized some of these things around his house might help him think about good memories. He had a box with medals and pictures that he could look at every year around anniversaries. He took some of these pictures out and bought frames to display them. John also had yearly Christmas cards from some of their families and made a commitment to send cards back next year. When he asked for help from his family, his son suggested they sign up for an annual charity event that supported other veterans.

As he worked on these elements, John noticed he was able to recall more of the positive memories he had forgotten. He wrote some of these down, which helped him recognize them and balance out negative memories. John then started to see how changing what he chose to dream about in rescription meant he could still think about his friends. After working through these exercises, John still believed he needed to have nightmares to honor his friends' memories, but he also thought that his friends would probably want him to have a better quality of life. Reducing the impact of nightmares on his sleep was a part of his recovery from trauma. Sleeping better gave him a clearer head and more energy to put toward valued activities.

Trauma survivors might find that when negative memories come up in the day or in nightmares, it seems to invite more negative memories. It can be hard to recall the positive events or even more neutral events when you are struggling with sleep and nightmares. Spending time trying to come up with positive events, while also working on reducing the nightmares, can help you gain a more balanced perspective. To get started with this tool, consider the following steps:

1. Tracking thoughts about sleep and nightmares

2. Looking for evidence for and against these thoughts

3. Making changes so the thoughts are more helpful or realistic

4. Creating and practicing new thoughts about sleep

5. Noticing how the new thought impacts your sleep

CHAPTER 12

Relapse Prevention

Congratulations on making it to this final chapter! Across this book, we challenged you to complete some difficult tasks. Here, we'll review the progress you have made, the skills you have learned, and share how to maintain or build upon your gains.

We introduced a lot of skills for responding to nightmares and sleep difficulties. You learned about healthy sleep and how nightmares and sleep problems develop in the first two chapters. Let's start by reviewing those points.

Sleep is a biological drive. Sleep is a two-process model involving the sleep drive and the circadian rhythm. We cannot make sleep happen, but we can influence how likely it is to happen by keeping regular bedtimes and wake times, and working on other elements that promote sleep like light exposure and managing hyperarousal.

Nightmares are learned behaviors. Therefore, they can be changed. Nightmares occur when the visual and emotional centers of our brain provide imagery to match how we feel. They can become a habit where the brain reaches for similar distressing content each night. People often escape nightmares through awakenings, which worsens sleep and next-day functioning—making nightmares more likely. Nightmares become a cycle:

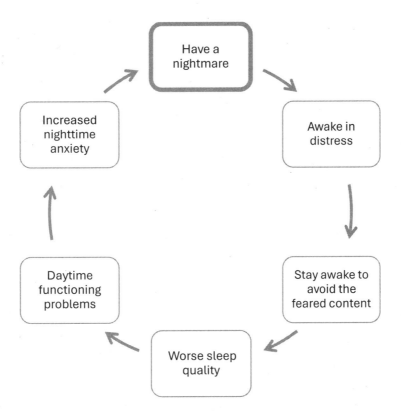

You can interrupt the cycle at multiple points using cognitive behavioral skills. Throughout this book, you have also learned evidence-based strategies for addressing nightmares and sleep problems through your targeted recovery plan. You may have chosen to read and implement strategies from every chapter or you may have been selective. At any time, you can return to those skills or add new ones from these chapters.

Skill	How to Use It
Sleep Tracking	Writing down information about your sleep and nightmares each morning to see key patterns and places for intervention.
Sleep Hygiene	Sleeping dos and don'ts that help ensure you are primed to sleep.
Relaxation	Breathing and progressive muscle relaxation skills that can reduce anxiety.
Visualization	Creating vivid mental pictures in your mind to hopefully get that information into your dreams.
Exposure	Approaching the feared nightmare content while awake through writing, which gives you more power over the nightmare to look for ways to change it.
Scripting and Rescription	Creating a new dream that you would like to dream using vivid imagery or altering the nightmare to create a new version that is pleasant or neutral.
Sleep Restriction	Limiting the time you spend in bed to the amount of sleep you can generate may help reduce insomnia.
Stimulus Control	Limiting your bed activities to sleep and sex to associate your bed with being asleep and not being awake.
Cognitive Restructuring	Finding thoughts that interfere with sleep and examining how helpful or realistic they are, and then changing these thoughts to more helpful thoughts.
Lucidity Checks	Testing yourself throughout the day to see if you're asleep encourages you to check during dreams so you become aware that you are dreaming and can change your dream while you have it.

Reviewing Your Progress

How are you doing with your goals? In the following table, write down your key goals and take a few minutes to rate them using a 0 to 100 scale. For this table, 0 may be where you started with this book or the worst point of your symptoms. A 100 would indicate your goal has been completely met. Considering where you started and where you would like to be, are you 0, 25, 50, 75, or 100 percent of the way there? Most people have a range for different goals. That's okay! You'll likely see improvement over time if you keep using the skills you have learned in this book.

Goal	Progress Toward Goal (0 to 100 percent)

Maybe you met all your goals, or you are just starting to see progress. Often change happens slowly over time. This is a reason we asked you to continue your sleep and nightmare logs. If you look at your logs from the first week or two of tracking compared to now, what differences do you see?

_____

_____

_____

_____

_____

How has your overall sleep improved?

_____
_____
_____
_____

Have your nightmares decreased in intensity, severity, frequency, or maybe even disappeared?

_____
_____
_____
_____

If you chose rescription, are you starting to have your new dream more often? Has the nightmare changed?

_____
_____
_____
_____

If you are seeing changes, it's helpful to consider what helped you to make those changes. Write down the elements of this program you have found most helpful. You'll then use this to create your relapse prevention plan.

Change in Sleep and Nightmares	Elements That Helped with This Change

Maintaining or Growing Your Recovery

Many people who found recovery from their nightmares have some doubts about their recovery. They worry that nightmares may return or that they won't be able to keep up the gains over time. We've found that if you use the skills in this book and you have practiced for long enough, you'll see the target nightmare change in intensity, frequency, or even disappear. You can usually trust that recovery after several weeks. We encourage you to continue practicing the new dream twice a day, for about a month.

Reflect on the areas where you would like to continue to grow your recovery and the elements you are committed to practicing. You should also set a time for this practice so you can reevaluate how the practice is working or not working.

Continued Growth Areas	Skills to Keep Practicing	Time I Commit to Doing This
Reducing the nightmare	Rescription	Continue twice daily practice of my new dream for two weeks.

The charts you have filled in across this chapter now become your recovery plan. You have reflected on your achievements, the skills that have been helpful, and the areas you need to continue to practice. We also want to take a moment to think about relapse prevention!

Relapse Prevention

We know that insomnia, sleep problems, and nightmares can return—especially in times of high stress. This can be good stress or bad stress! An example of good stressors might be something exciting like starting a new job or relationship, moving, or even having a new baby. Bad stressors could include medical challenges, difficulty in relationships, losses, or worsening mental health symptoms. Stressors can cause disruptions in our sleep for one night or several, but our sleep will usually bounce back.

If you notice difficulties with your sleep, we encourage you to track the sleep for one to two weeks. As you reflect on the tracking, do you notice that the disruption was temporary or is it sustained?

When we experience life stressors, we often stop doing the things that keep us on a regular schedule in sleep and life. One of the first recommendations is to prioritize bedtime and wake time, regular meals, and light exposure. Remember, getting pulled off your sleep rhythm or circadian rhythm can put you at higher risk! Trying to compensate for changes in sleep—like napping, spending more time in bed, or delaying sleep to avoid nightmares—increases your risk. Work first on stabilizing the sleep rhythm and attending to feelings of distress both at bedtime and during the day. Prioritize your favorite relaxation strategy to interrupt the nightmare cycle. It's likely good for addressing whatever stressor you are facing also.

If you're doing these things and still noticing difficulty, return to the other skills in this book that helped you. You may have temporary increases in symptoms, and sometimes those increases can be sustained, especially if you stop using your skills. Because nightmares are learned behavior, changing your behaviors can help prevent a few bad nights of sleep from becoming a more sustained nightmare problem. If you are noticing nightmares when tracking sleep changes in response to stressors, pay attention to what might be feeding the nightmare. Look for behaviors that might make the nightmares more frequent or intense. You can then identify which skills you need to focus on to address the relapse.

Final Thoughts

Nightmares are a challenging problem! Sleep and dreaming are basic biological needs, but when things are off track, it causes disruptions all twenty-four hours of the day. Recovery from nightmares does not mean you will have perfect sleep for the remainder of your life. Even healthy sleepers have an off night here and there. However, recovery from nightmares means you are in a place where nightmares no longer interfere with your daily life. Now that you've completed this book, you have a toolkit stocked with powerful strategies to help you move forward in life.

One of the most frequent questions asked when someone has completed sleep treatment is: "Do I still have to keep a steady bedtime and wake time?" As an adult, you can choose when you sleep. However, for most people, keeping to a healthy rhythm, especially the wake time, will keep their health in check and their sleep health in check too.

References

Benito, K. G., and Walther, M. (2015). Therapeutic process during exposure: Habituation model. *Journal of Obsessive-Compulsive and Related Disorders*, *6*, 147-157. https://doi.org/10.1016/j.jocrd.2015.01.006.

DeMarni Cromer, L., Pangelinan, B. A., and Buck, T. R. (2022). Case study of cognitive behavioral therapy for nightmares in children with and without trauma history. *Clinical Case Studies*, *21*(5), 377–395.

Mallett, R., Picard-Deland, C., Pigeon, W., Wary, M., Grewal, A., Blagrove, M., et al. (2021). The relationship between dreams and subsequent morning mood using self-reports and text analysis. *Affective Science*, 3(2), 400–405. https://doi.org/10.1007/s42761-021-00080-8.

Manconi, M., Ferri, R., Sargrada, C., Punjabi, N.M., Tettamanzi, E., Zucconi, M., Olandi, A., Castronovo, V. and Ferini-Strambi, L. (2010). Measuring the error in sleep estimation in normal subjects and in patients with insomnia. *Journal of Sleep Research*, *19*(3), 478–486. https://doi.org/10.1111/j.1365-2869.2009.00801.x.

Ouchene, R., El Habchi, N., Demina, A., Petit, B., and Trojak, B. (2023). The effectiveness of lucid dreaming therapy in patients with nightmares: A systematic review. *L'Encéphale*, *49*(5), 525–531.

Porter, K. M. (2003). *The Mental Athlete*. Human Kinetics.

Resick, P., Wiltsey Stirman, S., and LoSavio, S. T. (2023). *Getting Unstuck from PTSD: Using Cognitive Processing Therapy to Guide Your Recovery*. Guilford Press.

Sewart, A. R. and Craske, M. G. (2020). Inhibitory learning. In J. S. Abramowitz and S. M. Blakey (Eds.), *Clinical Handbook of Fear and Anxiety: Maintenance Processes and Treatment Mechanisms*, 265–285. American Psychological Association. https://doi.org/10.1037/0000150-015.

Courtney Worley, PhD, MPH, is a diplomate in behavioral sleep medicine, and board-certified clinical psychologist specializing in evidence-based interventions for sleep and trauma. Worley previously led the national implementation of written exposure therapy in the Department of Veterans Affairs (VA) as a system-wide training program. In her clinical practice at Upward Behavioral Health, she provides virtual services across the United States using evidence-based psychotherapies, including specialized sleep interventions and psychotherapies for post-traumatic stress disorder (PTSD). She serves as a trainer and consultant in the United States and internationally for clinicians and health care systems implementing evidence-based psychotherapies for PTSD. Her sleep research program includes investigating nightmare epidemiology and the comorbidity between nightmares and other psychiatric disorders.

Michael R. Nadorff, PhD, is professor of psychology at Mississippi State University. He completed a nightmare treatment study as his dissertation project, and has worked in nightmare treatment for well over a decade. His research focuses on the association between nightmares, as well as other sleep difficulties, and suicidal behavior. Nadorff has published more than one hundred peer-reviewed manuscripts, and has been cited more than 4,700 times. He has received more than fifteen million dollars in grant funding, with active external grant awards from NIMH, SAMHSA, and the CDC. He is also past president of the Society of Behavioral Sleep Medicine.

Foreword writer **Brigitte Holzinger, PhD,** is a clinical and health psychologist, licensed teacher, psychotherapist, sleep coach, and licensed somnologist (ESRS). Her research focuses on sleep, dreams, lucid dreaming, and nightmares. Holzinger cofounded the Austrian Sleep Research Association (ASRA) and the Institute for Consciousness and Dream Research (ICDR) in Vienna, Austria.

Real change *is* possible

For more than fifty years, New Harbinger has published proven-effective self-help books and pioneering workbooks to help readers of all ages and backgrounds improve mental health and well-being, and achieve lasting personal growth. In addition, our spirituality books offer profound guidance for deepening awareness and cultivating healing, self-discovery, and fulfillment.

Founded by psychologist Matthew McKay and Patrick Fanning, New Harbinger is proud to be an independent, employee-owned company. Our books reflect our core values of integrity, innovation, commitment, sustainability, compassion, and trust. Written by leaders in the field and recommended by therapists worldwide, New Harbinger books are practical, accessible, and provide real tools for real change.

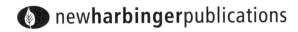

MORE BOOKS from
NEW HARBINGER PUBLICATIONS

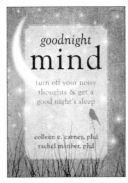

GOODNIGHT MIND

Turn Off Your Noisy Thoughts and Get a Good Night's Sleep

978-1608826186 / US $21.95

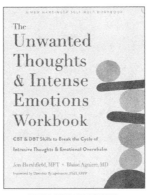

THE UNWANTED THOUGHTS AND INTENSE EMOTIONS WORKBOOK

CBT and DBT Skills to Break the Cycle of Intrusive Thoughts and Emotional Overwhelm

978-1648480553 / US $24.95

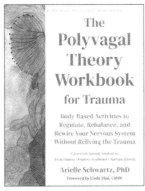

THE POLYVAGAL THEORY WORKBOOK FOR TRAUMA

Body-Based Activities to Regulate, Rebalance, and Rewire Your Nervous System Without Reliving the Trauma

978-1648484162 / US $25.95

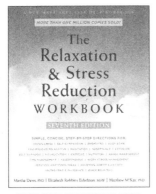

THE RELAXATION AND STRESS REDUCTION WORKBOOK, SEVENTH EDITION

978-1684033348 / US $28.95

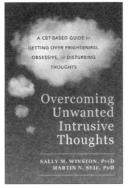

OVERCOMING UNWANTED INTRUSIVE THOUGHTS

A CBT-Based Guide to Getting Over Frightening, Obsessive, or Disturbing Thoughts

978-1626254343 / US $18.95

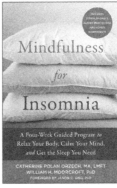

MINDFULNESS FOR INSOMNIA

A Four-Week Guided Program to Relax Your Body, Calm Your Mind, and Get the Sleep You Need

978-1684032587 / US $25.95

newharbingerpublications

1-800-748-6273 / newharbinger.com

(VISA, MC, AMEX / prices subject to change without notice)

Follow Us

Don't miss out on new books from New Harbinger.
Subscribe to our email list at **newharbinger.com/subscribe**

Did you know there are **free tools** you can download for this book?

Free tools are things like **worksheets**, **guided meditation exercises**, and **more** that will help you get the most out of your book.

You can download free tools for this book—whether you bought or borrowed it, in any format, from any source—from the New Harbinger website. All you need is a NewHarbinger.com account. Just use the URL provided in this book to view the free tools that are available for it. Then, click on the "download" button for the free tool you want, and follow the prompts that appear to log in to your NewHarbinger.com account and download the material.

You can also save the free tools for this book to your **Free Tools Library** so you can access them again anytime, just by logging in to your account! Just look for this button on the book's free tools page.

+ Save this to my free tools library

If you need help accessing or downloading free tools, visit **newharbinger.com/faq** or contact us at **customerservice@newharbinger.com**.